Entering an online support group on eating disorders

Utrecht Studies in Language and Communication

21

Entering an online support group on eating disorders

A discourse analysis

Wyke Stommel

Amsterdam - New York, NY 2009

Cover art: Shirley Hartlage

The paper on which this book is printed meets the requirements of "ISO 9706:1994, Information and documentation - Paper for documents - Requirements for permanence".

ISBN: 978-90-420-2660-5
E-Book ISBN: 978-90-420-2661-2

Printed in The Netherlands

Table of contents

Part II – Discourse analysis

Acknowledgements

Many people have supported me in the process of writing this thesis. I would like to thank Tom Koole for his supervision of the study from beginning to end. He helped me to develop the ideas, critically commented on the analyses and wisely advised me when I came to him with various academic questions. He helped me keep my focus, despite of the fact that I switched universities and disciplines. I also want to thank Katharina Liebsch for her supervision of my work over the past two years. Thanks to her, I have been able to finish my sociology Ph.D. I thank Marlis Hellinger of the linguistics department for her useful comments on the early drafts of parts of this thesis.

My research was only made possible because of the financial support I received from the Marie Curie Fellowship. Therefore, I thank the European Union for its generous facilitation of my research. I am very grateful to Brita Rang, who managed the scholarship issues at Frankfurt University. She made me feel welcome in Frankfurt from the minute I arrived and advised me in both research and personal matters during the three years I spent there. I also participated in the Frankfurt and Kassel Interdisciplinary Training Group "Public Spheres and Gender Relations: Dimensions of Experience." I thank all of the members of this group, including both the professors and fellow Ph.D. students for the exciting discussions on gender, methodology and theoretical issues. My gender awareness has grown substantially thanks to them.

Some of my colleagues at Frankfurt University deserve special thanks for their valuable contributions to my work. First of all, I thank Fabienne Imlinger, who commented on practically every aspect of my text over the past two years. We intensely discussed research issues again and again, which has definitely made me a better scholar. Moreover, I am very grateful for the friendship that has developed between us. Second, I received many sharp observations and good ideas during the data sessions with Verena Haug, Juliane Hogrefe, Nils Köbel, Meron Mendel and Jessica Weil. Thank you!

If Hungrig-Online had not given me permission to observe their forum, this thesis would not have been written. Therefore, I am very grateful to the members of Hungrig-Online who gave their permission for me to use their contributions and/or nicknames for the analysis. Their discussions, which often consisted of the very first words they typed in the forum, have enabled me to develop the insights that I present in this thesis. I sincerely hope that the Hungrig-Online community benefits from my study. Moreover, I thank Wolfgang Gawlik and Birte Zess, from the Hungrig-Online staff, who were always ready to explain things about the forum, and even commented on several of my chapters.

Some people have cooperated professionally on several issues related to this book. I thank Torsten Kutschke for his view on the juridical question regarding Internet research and German law, Thomas Gloning (Marburg University) for his thoughts on the research proposal in its earliest stage, Christel Vierboom and Greet Kuipers for explaining eating disorders to me, Reinhold Schmitt and his colleagues from the *Institut für Deutsche Sprache* in Mannheim for the inspiring data sessions, Joyce Lamerichs for commenting on various analyses, Millie Baker for her translations of the Hungrig-Online excerpts and Bart Plantenga for the proofreading.

I thank my parents, brother and friends for their continued support in my academic efforts and beyond.

At about the halfway point in writing this book, a very special person entered my life. I thank Timo for standing by me, since that very first day in October 2006. And finally, I thank Charlotte, because she enabled me to write a substantial part of this book, while I was carrying her.

Introduction

Imagine the following situation. Despite your attempts to ignore it, you know that you have a serious problem. You consider joining an online support group to get in touch with others who understand what you're going through, possibly even better than you, and who may even be able to offer their help. You search a forum in your own language and read a few contributions to check whether it appeals to you. You decide to register, check off the Rules and Regulations and try to come up with a nickname that has not been registered yet, and, more importantly, one that suits you. You receive a password and wonder how to actually get started in this forum. You decide to post a contribution in the sub-forum for new members to introduce yourself and see how the other members react to your story. How should you present yourself? What is one allowed to tell, and what is not allowed? Is your condition even bad enough to participate in the first place? You also feel nervous because you have seldom told anyone about your problem, but you collect all the courage necessary and post your first message. A couple of hours later you receive an answer; a respondent welcomes you, reassures you that you have found the right place to discuss your concerns and she briefly tells you something about herself. You feel relieved, but also anxious; you are in.

The above-described phenomenon of entering an online support group is the topic of investigation of this book. Although the web-based services of forums and support groups have the appearance of being low-threshold, the actual steps involved in becoming an active participant in a forum can be quite difficult. Presumably, the threshold of entering is partly dependent on the role other members of the online forum play in response to new members' first contributions. What really seems to matter is the extent to which members perceive and treat the forum (population) as a community. If the number of active participants is high enough, a certain sense of community can arise from an online venue, not only in playful environments such as virtual worlds and games, but also in problem-oriented environments such as online support groups. This study thus attempts to shed light on how an online forum, which enables the coming together of a group of people with a specific affliction, works and what role it plays in illness behavior. One highly relevant aspect of the community-phenomenon in online support groups I focus on is the interactive practice of entering a forum to become a member, and the extent to which this process is characterized by patterns or regularities, which imply a certain normatively appropriate behavior.

Nowadays, online support group services are innumerable. Research on such groups is always confronted with the question to what extent the phenomena are specific for the type of affliction the forum is devoted to. The present study focuses an online forum on eating disorders. Despite the (mental) particularities of these disorders, the study does not put eating disorders as such in focus, but aims to analyze processes of online support groups that may play a role in groups on other psychiatric conditions as well. Theoretically, the step to join an online support group is therefore interpreted as the adoption of the sick role (Parsons, 1951), which is difficult for all psychiatric syndromes, in part due to the stigma tied to them.

Still, a study of an online support group on eating disorders must be placed in the wider context of eating disorders. The members of the online support group under investigation are predominantly adolescent women struggling with anorexia and/or bulimia. Anorexia, characterized by the persistence of the sufferer's refusal to eat, is all about being very, very thin, while bulimia is characterized by its more clandestine nature of the survival mechanism that involves gorging and purging as a way to not have to pay (i.e., gain weight) for what is perceived as greed (Orbach, 1993). Many sufferers go through bulimic and anorectic stages in alternation, along with phases of compulsive overeating. In 1993, Orbach noted that one of the barriers to the development of prevention and treatment programs for the hundreds of thousands of individual women with eating problems was a "lack of collective engagement … that keeps their problems hidden, unrecognized and inadequately considered" (1993: xxiv). With the steady rise of Internet availability, it appears that, since 1993, people with eating problems have also found a virtual locus where they can openly share and discuss their concerns. A lot of media attention has been paid to so-called "pro-ana" (pro-anorexia) and "pro-mia" (pro-bulimia) websites, blogs and forums, which contradict the dominant medical perceptions of how to treat eating disorders as they celebrate the disorders as a preferred lifestyle. Very little public attention has been paid to web-based environments that specifically criticize the promotion of the proliferation of eating disorders. These forums offer a primary alternative to the isolation in which mostly girls struggle with weight and food, and encourage them to seek professional help. This study engages an example of the latter type of online forum, one that belongs to the German Web site *Hungrig-Online* (HO).

The issue of mental disorders such as eating disorders is a sensitive one, partly due to shame, and this offers an indication that joining an online forum like this may not be without its problems. The topic of entering an online support group is therefore intricately connected to the characteristics of eating disorders. Joining HO is frequently the first step girls take to disclose something about their problems, hence, a highly delicate undertaking. The other members recognize the amount of courage that was probably required to actually make that initial contact and they show their appreciation, even if the new member has come up with some dubious feelings or thoughts regarding eating behavior and body perception. The members tend to ignore these potentially "dangerous" ideas in the interest of being helpful. The present study will offer a microanalysis of these prickly activities, which must be considered the essential first steps on the difficult path to recovery.

The most important research aim of this study is to provide a description of the social aspects of entering an online support group related to the categories of community and identity. It is analyzed how these categories point to norms that are relevant for becoming a member of this group. This includes the following issues:

- The type of nicknames members use and how they depict personal characteristics.
- The relevance of the legitimacy for joining the forum and how it is communicated.
- The modes in which novices present themselves and their affliction in their first posting.
- The means by which newcomers are accepted or rejected by regular members.
- The display of community or the orientation towards being a community.

Furthermore, I embed the empirical phenomena inside a larger theoretical framework on illness behavior. The ways members present their illness and the norms of membership, as they are relevant in the forum interactions can be interpreted as sick role behavior (Parsons, 1951).

The chosen approach for the empirical part is a discourse analysis of chains of contributions by novice members and the HO-forum's regular members. The analytical focus is on "doing community" and "doing identity" in these interactions. I approach the concepts of community and identity from a discursive point of view, with a strong emphasis on ethnomethodology and Conversation Analysis. The focus is on observable discourse, which means that interpretations of discourse that are of a cognitive, psychological, or other nature have been avoided. The central question is how participants, through their online messages, accomplish actions and display their understanding of one another's actions, and whether and how these actions relate to one another.

In general, both sociological and linguistic research interests and theories have informed and guided the analysis, implying that this study is a product of an interdisciplinary research conduct. For discourse analysts in the field of linguistics, the study is important with regard to the issue of CMC (computer-mediated communication) in general and, more specifically, the question of how members communicate particular interests and identities. For instance, the observation that novice members somehow express an insecure or uncertain attitude in relation to the forum demands a description of how insecurity is discursively articulated and also leads to the question of what "performed" insecurity accomplishes in an interactional setting. The general interactional pattern seems to be that insecure openings stimulate welcomes in response, but also that the employment of various oral discourse features helps construct an ambivalent position in relation to the addressees.

Another example in which the relevance of discourse is important in the present study is the issue of accountability for a certain state of being, namely mental illness such as an eating disorder. The discursive construction of (accounts of) mental illness has received quite a lot of research attention, but hitherto, primarily transcripts of encounters of the ill with the healthy (mostly interviewers and doctors) have been analyzed. The present analysis of the discursive construction of mental illness vis-à-vis a peer community thus yields new insights in the field of discourse analysis, such as the role of one's knowledge about the illness, displayed by the use of medical terminology.

For sociologists, the summarized research objectives are particularly interesting from a medical-sociological perspective. The rise of online support groups can be viewed as a phenomenon related to the increase in individual responsibility for health and related self-observation and self-help issues. I attempt to address the question of how these groups are related to the general social norms relevant to being ill (i.e., the *sick role*). With regard to eating disorders, the pro-ana development embodies the break with, or threat to medically dominant approaches to illness as an involuntary state of being that requires professional treatment. Hence, the medically dominant norms (that are incorporated into diagnostic models) are challenged here. The question the study addresses is to what extent peer, lay online support groups actually subscribe to the sick role's norms. It is revealed that upon entering the forum, the sick role's norms are relaxed since the regular members seem to prioritize the social interest involved in including new members in the community.

The book is divided into roughly three parts. In part 1, I lay out the theoretical foundations of the study. I consider various concepts of community and identity, which have been used in previous research (both linguistic and social scientific) and select approaches that serve an ethnomethodological study of online community and connected identities (chapter 1.1 and 1.2). As a result, both community and identity are seen as discursive accomplishments rather than objectively observable, subjective or cognitive entities. Chapter 1.3 focuses on the topic of the online support group that the analysis is dedicated to: eating disorders. I approach eating disorders as social phenomena, which includes an examination of diagnostic criteria and the role of stigma. I refrain from assuming that the participants in online support groups are medically diagnosed as having eating disorders, but prefer to characterize *being eating disordered* as an identity, which requires discursive articulation like any other identity that is assumed in an online environment.

In part 2, I begin by introducing the methodical issues relevant to the study, among which, an elaborate consideration of the ethics involved in using sensitive research material. The main features of Discourse Analysis and Conversation Analysis as I use them are introduced here as well. Subsequently, the findings of the Discourse Analysis are presented in four chapters.

Chapter 2.2 begins by presenting an analysis of the nicknames used by members. Nicknames are important to consider, because the choice of a nickname is an unavoidable step in the process of entering the online support group and because these nicknames often exhibit various personal traits of the individual forum members, which can tell us something about who these members are. In chapter 2.3, I analyze how novice members open their first posts to the forum. What is important here are the discursive/interactional features such as features of oral language use and the way that certain characteristics of introductory postings typically seem to call up a specific type of response. Chapter 2.4 focuses on the various fashions cited by novice members to account for their presence in the forum, hence, the display of *forumability*, and the way regular members accept these accounts with (more or less) identification and cordiality. Chapter 2.5 is also dedicated to forumability, but here I focus on the threads initiated by novice members who are unsure about whether they even have an eating disorder, or who are in denial about their being ill, which sometimes leads to friction with regular members.

In the final part (3), the findings are considered with regard to the question of how the communicative behavior in the online support groups relates to the sick role (Parsons, 1951; Suchman, 1965; Mechanic, 1978). Many newcomers to the online support group appear to find themselves in the early stages of the sick role. Entering the group is treated as a great step in the direction of accepting the affliction and thus adoption of the sick role. However, the sick role as a theoretical concept requires some adaption to take account of this process.

Part I

An ethnomethodological approach to community, identity and eating disorders

Chapter 1

The online support group as a community

1.1 Introduction

The importance of web-based communities in people's everyday lives has grown rapidly since the early 1990s. More and more "wired" individuals are involved in various online environments, such as mailing lists, newsgroups, newsboards (forums), IRC-channels (chat) and MUDs.[1] Social relationships are created and maintained at and through these virtual locations. However, despite the development of visual and audio technologies (such as webcams and podcasts), a large part of the activity in most online communities remains text-based, i.e., communication is restricted to typed text and predetermined graphics (mainly smileys or emoticons). This means that the primary activity in online communities is type-written computer-mediated communication (CMC).

Along with the rise of online communities, the research interests in what actually happens there, how these communities are built or structured, how the communications between members can be characterized, how individuals experience life online, etc. is increasing. In the 1990s, research on virtual communities paid more attention to the liberating or democratic aspects of virtual life facilitated by the technical and textual character of the medium. Social relationships in online environments were the main focus of attention for the, by now classical, studies of the community called The WELL (Rheingold, 2000) and the psychology of online life (Turkle, 1995). Virtual communities were declared beneficial for personal well-being, but also ascribed the power to subvert the stringent, deeply inscribed rules of social life (gender, ethnicity, sexuality, disability, etc.). Thus, virtual communities were celebrated for their liberating and progressive potential. Some years later, however, this view began to be criticized as a kind of postmodern utopianism (Sundèn, 2003; Yates, 1997). It was eventually discovered that the actual swapping of identities or the playing of fictional roles online was extremely rare, since

---

[1] A MUD is a text-based environment that allows a large number of people to connect to it and provides each user access to this virtual world by using a simple programming language, which enables them to manipulate the database from the 'inside' and build or add 'rooms' and other objects. A MUD is a kind of virtual reality, an electronically represented text-only space that users can visit.

most users do not remain anonymous for very long, using signatures or nicknames as authentic self presentations (Döring, 2003; Misoch, 2004). In line with this, Kennedy has claimed that "the time has come for Internet identity research to reposition itself conceptually, to move away from a preoccupation with the generalized, enduring claim that Internet identities are anonymous, multiple and fragmented" (2006: 859) and, instead, consider offline and online identities in relation to one another. It is only when people want to discuss socially sensitive issues that they opt for anonymity, but not with the intention of deceiving others or transgressing their offline identities. An important factor in this involves the type of online community the user accesses. This ranges from role-playing online to discussion boards on political or health-related issues. Thus, recent studies have begun to recognize that different types of virtual communities need to be distinguished (e.g., Herring, 2008 in press), including interest groups (e.g., soap opera fans), support groups (health-related), task-related groups (education), geographically based groups and commercial environments.

In this chapter, I focus on the relationship between health- or illness-related support groups and virtual or online communities. First, however, I will investigate the frequently heard beneficial aspects of online support groups (1.2). Section 1.3 explains how some studies implicitly suggest that community aspects, such as legitimacy, are, in fact, relevant in online support groups, possibly influencing their beneficial effects. However, the concept of community should not be used uncritically; section 1.4 investigates the debate surrounding the use of the concept of (online/virtual) community as opposed to group. In the search for a useful empirical definition of community, I review previous studies of online communities (1.5). They are reviewed for their conceptualization of community, which is either a priori defined in terms of criteria or based on a feeling or sense of community. I propose an alternative view by considering the online community from an ethnomethodological perspective, which means that the focus is on the participants' accomplishments of community. Section 1.6 argues that the concept of Community of Practice (CoP) offers the framework to facilitate an ethnomethodological/interactional approach without losing sight of the external structures such as technical limits and forum guidelines.

1.2 The benefits of online support groups

Previous research has mapped out the advantages of online groups, usually through the use of questionnaires. The most frequently heard advantages include 24-hour availability, geographic independence, selective participation in reading and responding to messages, anonymity and privacy, and immediate and/or delayed responses (Döring, 1997). Moreover, it is noted that writing allows thoughts to be formed more slowly and edited more carefully and that personal triumphs seem clearer and more powerful in the written word than in real life encounters (King, 1994). Hence, special benefits are ascribed to the characteristics of written communication.

An advantage of a different kind is the phenomenon of *lurking*, which refers to the fact that the majority of "members" of online groups are solely readers or spectators, i.e., they do not contribute any input themselves (Preece et al., 2004; M. Smith and Kollock, 1999).[2] This is considered a virtue, especially in the case of online support groups, since these silent members are unlikely to join face-to-face self-help groups because they feel shame, embarrassment or have other inhibitions. But online they can have access to the narratives, the advice and experiences of other sufferers. The feeling of "I am not alone" is thus not only a positive effect of active participation, but also of lurking. Therefore, the option of lurking without having to reveal oneself is considered a positive trait. The disadvantage, however, is that if (lurking) members withdraw from the virtual community for whatever reason (being hurt or shocked by a posting or undergoing a relapse), the online support group has no indication of this, unlike in face-to-face groups, and thus cannot offer a safety net.

Research on the potential beneficial (e.g., informative, supportive, therapeutic) effects of the Internet as a source of social support and health information is increasing rapidly (e.g., Burrows et al., 2000; King, 1994; Lasker et al., 2005; Loader et al., 2002). Health-related searches have become one of the top three uses of the Internet (Brann and Anderson, 2002) and the leading source of information is from support groups that link people with common problems together (Cotten and Gupta, 2004). In addition to the exchange of medical information, interaction with others with similar conditions enables people to share their experiences and emotional support. Some studies suggest that the dominant reason of the two (either sharing biomedical information or support) in a certain group depends on the problem: In an Alzheimer's mail group, seeking and offering information dominated, while in another group devoted to the disabled, socio-emotional interaction dominated. However, others found that it depended on gender: In cancer support groups women were more likely to offer their support and encouragement, while

[2] The phenomenon of lurking raises the question of whether lurkers should be called members of the community. According to one definition, a group is a community when membership is consequential, which means that when a member fails to show up, it may be noted and addressed (i.e., it has consequences) by the community (Opielka, 2004). Thus, this definition excludes lurkers from the community. Still, lurking must be seen as a positive side effect of online support groups.

men were more likely to communicate information (Lasker et al., 2005). In conclusion, however, both information and support seem to be of interest to users of online support groups. In effect, participation in an online group helps people suffering from cancer (Schultz, 2002), disabilities (Finn, 1999), depression (Galegher et al., 1998) and many other problems in dealing with coping.

Helping others cope with a problem can be seen as a positive addition to the professional medical treatment of a particular condition (Binik et al., 1997). For example, in groups for addicts, the benefits go beyond support and information seeking/providing, as they may actually aid in a participant's recovery. King (1994) sought to determine, through questionnaires, if the involvement in a support group for alcoholics improved the alcoholics' chances of recovery. The results showed that it did. Getting and giving emotional support seemed to complement their attendance of meetings and other recovery methods. Moreover, the longer they tended to participate, the more they appeared to benefit, since participation included activities usually associated with close friendships. King claimed that addiction, unlike other medical conditions, often depends on peer support for any particular program to be successful. Therefore,

> [a]ddicts who exchange stories, information and emotional support by computers are not just engaged in an adjunct to their therapy, [but] that activity is part of their therapy (1994: 51).

In an interview, one of the participants explained that some of the members became good friends and that he missed them now that they had left the group. Hence, this study allows us to surmise that the social relationships in online support groups may have a therapeutic value, particularly among groups for addicts, such as alcoholics, but potentially also for sufferers of other addictions. This means that online support groups, in spite of or because of their textual character, are not only important as a medium for information exchange and support, but also for their therapeutic effects on the people with severe problems.

1.3 The role of community aspects in online support groups

Despite their beneficial effects, it has been observed that online support groups have high dropout rates (Sandaunet, 2008), hence, these groups are not successful in every respect. It could be that members withdraw from the group due to specific CMC phenomena. In the early days of CMC research, flaming in web-based groups was seen as a typical CMC phenomenon and explained by the reduced availability of social cues (Kiesler et al., 1984). However, this hypothesis was rejected by other studies that revealed that uninhibited behavior is not dependent on, or inherent to the medium, but instead takes place in a social context that is pre-defined or communicated via the medium (e.g., Höflich, 1996; Lea et al., 1992). This supports the idea that social processes such as community aspects could play a role in dropout from online support groups. Sandaunet (2008) identified several conditions for non-participation or withdrawal from an online cancer self-help group, of which two are significant with respect to the community aspects of the group: One was not being "ill enough" to participate, and the second condition was the challenge of establishing a legitimate position in the group. It seems that participation in an online community requires legitimacy, which is related to the state of the illness and the position in the group, both of which are aspects of the member's identity. Galegher et al. explained the importance of displaying legitimacy in *face-to-face* groups and posed the question of how the members of *online* groups are able to display it under web-based conditions:

> To obtain direct support and information from others in the group, one must demonstrate legitimacy – that his or her concerns are genuine and justified. In a face-to-face support group, a member's physical presence at a meeting is usually sufficiently informative to legitimate that member's claim on the groups' attention. But the actions associated with showing up also reveal a more elaborated wish for legitimacy within the group. For example, one might, at a minimum, dress appropriately (albeit casually), travel to the group, wear a stick-on name tag regardless of the length of one's membership, and contribute to the coffee fund. These actions illustrate that the group and its conventions are important to the individual – that he or she wants to be a legitimate member of the group. This display of belongingness increases the likelihood that the individual will be granted some airtime while others will pay attention and respond when he or she speaks. ... What, then, do individuals in computer-mediated groups do to reveal their commitment, to ensure that their contributions will be seen as legitimate? (1998: 449-500).

The study these researchers conducted revealed that novice participants of online support groups, who did not explicitly legitimate their membership during their contributions, were likely to be ignored. Claims which serve to legitimate one's participation may involve the group itself (how long the poster has lurked before posting, or referring to other postings) or the group's membership (descriptions of symptoms or diagnosis). Galegher et al. (1998: 513) have stressed that the challenge of legitimacy may be particularly difficult for novice members. In general, the issue of legitimacy seems to be a precondition for the promising effect of online support groups.

There is another question regarding the causal relations between community aspects of online support groups and recovery: Do particularly community-like groups have a positive influence on recovery, or does peer interaction in a non-community environment have the same effect? Burrows et al. have contended that although online support groups in some ways are virtual communities, "they are nevertheless simply the result of a collection of contributions from individuals" (2000: 115). According to Williams (1989), individualism and collectivism come together in self-help groups, but individualism remains the dominant partner. Individualism is rooted in the exaltation of a certain independence from others and a sense of autonomy, which are basic aspects of self-help. However, this seems to be a short-sighted perception regarding the role of the collective or the community in support groups. In a publicly accessible support forum, the clear division between collectivism and individualism is problematic, because even when single individuals write to other individuals in an online setting, they always have a larger audience and the participation in discussions is open to all members. The potential importance of the community in these discussions should not a priori be subordinate to the individualistic character of self-help. In fact, it appears that interaction and multiple social relations go hand in hand (e.g., King, 1996), which can, in turn, have a positive influence on recovery. Moreover, it appears that legitimacy is a precondition for community membership (Galegher et al., 1998), which implies that online support groups can only be beneficial when people are accepted as legitimate members. The role the community aspects play in an online support group may thus not be deferred.

It appears however, that previous studies of online support groups do not investigate the role of community aspects. Burrows et al. (2000), who entitled their article "Virtual Community Care," have not specified how they perceive the concept of community. They state:

> Whether or not the large number of social actors who currently engage in online self-help and social support constitute themselves into virtual communities is a key area for debate .... But whatever conceptualization one favours there is no doubt that growing numbers of people across the globe are using e-mail, the World Wide Web, mailing and discussion lists, newsgroups, MUDs, IRC and other forms of computer mediated communication (CMC) to offer and receive information, advice and support across a massive range of health and social issues (Burrows et al., 2000: 101).

These authors observed that the virtual geography is in flux, which means that the trend is toward online self-help and support fusing with web pages and other systems of information. This is why they suggested that a definition of community has become superfluous.

Most studies of self-help in online support groups failed to study the role of the community per se (e.g., Lasker et al., 2005; Winzelberg, 1997). They collected material from an online platform and code postings for various categories. Loader et al. (2002), for instance, analyzed a Usenet group on diabetes and distinguished types of social support, coding threads (chains of interrelated messages) for five categories: Social companionship, esteem, instrumentality, information and rude and intimidating postings. Threads are coded for one category only, although in rare case they are scored for two categories. Alternatively, Lasker et al. (2005) did not score postings, but "acts" (i.e., sentences or thoughts) in the postings. When various levels of communication (sentences vs. threads) are coded, quantitative analysis is useful to come up with a general idea of what online forums are "used for" (roughly varying from support to information).

However, there are also various disadvantages to this kind of research. The first point of critique is that the analysis is based on the researchers' categories, which ignores the participants' categories. To put it differently, it could be that the concept "support" is not a term that participants use in their discussions, which renders the ascription of the attribute "supportive" to a thread or an act as debatable. The researcher decides whether a posting or "act" is supportive, without taking into account if and in what manner the addressee of the allegedly supportive message treats it as a supportive act. For instance, if someone describes his disease, and a recipient responds with a mutual narrative about his own disease, should we label this as supportive? It could also be considered rude to ignore the first person's story and immediately present one's personal story. In other words, it is precarious to score postings for predefined categories. Second, postings of support are coded as independent of location in the forum although there may be various sub-forums (e.g., writing that you have recovered from an addiction may be received differently in a sub-forum for recovered members than in the sub-forum for new members). Furthermore, textual units are coded without taking into account the issue of membership, i.e., which member has written what. The question of whether experienced members act differently than novice members is thus ignored, but also the possible relevance of the member's type or severity of his or her condition. According to Lasker et al. (2005), a task for future research would be to look more explicitly at the leadership in online group cultures. They have suggested that posts from more "senior" peer experts may provide role models for newer members. But these authors have not specified what approach would best serve this purpose.

1.4 Online support group = online community?

Scrutiny is required when labeling an online support group as a community. In mainstream sociological discourse, groups are categorized into various types. Some scholars have proposed definitions, criteria or concepts (e.g., Opielka, 2004). One classical approach distinguishes between formal and personal relationships, and between primary and secondary groups where primary and secondary refers to the "psychological" relevance of the group for the individual (Cooley, 1909; for the application to computer-mediated groups see Döring, 2003). Primary groups with a certain level of socio-emotional relations are then called a community. An example is that of therapy groups, which should be considered formal primary groups, which in turn means that they are formally constituted (as opposed to family) and subjectively, highly regarded by the individual.

At the same time, it must also be recognized that each member may value the group differently, which means that the subjective perspective of the members should also be considered. Because of the connotations of *community* such as warmth and intimacy, Döring (2003: 491) has defined a therapy group as more than just a formal primary group, preferring the therapy *community* concept. Some studies of computer-mediated support forums, newsgroups, etc., called them virtual *communities* (e.g., Burrows et al., 2000; Loader et al., 2002), while other studies preferred support *groups* (e.g., Galegher et al., 1998; King, 1994; Lamerichs, 2003).

Although a definition has already been suggested with regard to groups versus communities, it seems that the distinction is not considered relevant in many empirical studies, and is more a matter of (the researcher's) own taste. We could thus conclude that it is irrelevant whether an online environment is called a community or something else, but this is not necessarily the case. Dyson (1997, cit. in Cherny, 1999) expressed her skepticism a decade ago about the use of the "C-word" since everyone uses it in slightly different ways. Moreover, others have disapproved of the inattentive distribution of the term community to various online conveniences. For instance, Döring (2003: 501) claimed that we should not label each online forum an online group, because a group implies not only a technical infrastructure, but moreover human members, group roles, social norms, etc. This renders the very loose definition of virtual community as a social group, whose members have met online and interact mainly through the Internet, questionable. Some other critics have, meanwhile, rejected the concept of community as applied to virtual groups altogether, because they considered it confusing in relation to the more traditional sociological uses of the word community or *Gemeinschaft* (Thiedeke, 2000). In other words, the concept *virtual/online community* has caused its share of disagreement among Internet researchers.

However, there is some consensus concerning the differences between online and offline groups or communities. It is generally agreed that technical facilitation (i.e., web-based, telephone, face-to-face) is less deterministic with regard to member types, group norms, etc. than the thematic focus. For instance, it can pretty much be assumed that an online self-help group is more similar to an offline self-help group than to an online trading community. An accurate comparison, however, is difficult to make, since today most social groups are actually hybrid groups, in which people have contact face-to-face, online and via other media, all combined in various proportions (Döring, 2003). A comparative study of hobby newsgroups and support newsgroups did confirm that these two types of groups exhibit different discourse styles with regard to legitimacy (legitimacy is saliently less important in hobby newsgroups), which suggests that the topic of the online group is more influential than the online/offline difference (Galegher et al., 1998). In other words, when the focus is on an online support group with a particular theme, the issue seems to be not the web-based modus of the group's communication, but the extent to which the group is an online community.

1.5 Defining community as an accomplishment

In contrast to studies of online support groups, studies of other types of online groups have explicitly considered the role of the community in online venues. They either looked at virtual community from an ethnographic point of view and then reflected upon it theoretically, or operationalized the concept of community before empirically studying it. Cherny (1999) reviewed various sociological and anthropological concepts of community in order to study the ElseMOO, a type of MUD. ElseMOO appeared to have features of a speech community, *community of memory*, social network, Community of Practice, etc. In her analysis, Cherny has used both "objective" features such as formal versus informal language use, network ties,[3] etc. and "subjective" features, such as personal feelings, or beliefs about the community: "The MUDders who frequent ElseMOO feel a strong sense of community identity" (1999: 267). With regard to community boundaries, a symbolic definition of community is referred to, which means that boundaries are in the minds of the members and the excluded (Cohen, 1985). Perceptions of boundaries may differ among individuals, and they are claimed to be dependent on abstractions such as friendship, rivalry, jealousy and similarity. Gossip was found to

[3] See also Stegbauer (2000), who argued that social structures can only be understood by analyzing the density of the communication, i.e., who interacts with whom, and how frequently. This is also an objective for social network analysis (Wellman, 1988,; 1997).

be a discursive (as opposed to a mental) issue in dealing with the community's boundaries. Virtual community is thus, according to Cherny, a phenomenon with characteristics of various (theories of) types of offline communities.

Herring (2004), in contrast to Cherny, has attempted to operationalize *community* in order to empirically analyze to what extent two online environments are virtual communities. For this purpose, she defined six sets of criteria, which characterize the concept of community:

1. An active, self-sustaining participation, a core of regular participants.
2. A shared history, purpose, culture, norms and values.
3. Solidarity, support, reciprocity.
4. Criticism, conflict, a means of conflict resolution.
5. Self-awareness of the group as an entity distinct from other groups.
6. Emergence of roles, hierarchy, governance, rituals.

According to Herring, each criterion, or level of analysis, requires its own method of analysis.[4] Nevertheless, she noted that the question of whether the extent of community-like behavior is sufficient to justify labeling an online environment a virtual community poses interpretive challenges. In fact, the establishment of objective criteria is necessarily arbitrary, and she therefore suggested that one must also take into account the perceptions of the participants themselves with regard to their own sense of community. Thus, Herring, like other researchers (e.g., Dubé et al., 2006; Korenman and Wyatt, 1996), believed community is "in the eye of the beholder" (i.e., the researcher), grounded in criteria, although it is recognized that community is also something subjective, a perception, an experience, a feeling that the *members* of the group have. Some empirical studies have taken this into account by using questionnaires in order to measure attitudes about the group. Korenman and Wyatt (1996), who studied group dynamics in a feminist email forum, proceeded in this twofold manner. They both relied on questionnaires filled out by users of the forum to find out how they experience the group, and studied discourse practices of the online group with the help of content analysis.

However, measuring attitudes through questionnaires has been criticized not only because of the problem of accurate representation (those who fill out the questionnaire are more likely to be active participants, than the general membership), but also because attitudes are not just in people's minds, but rather embedded in larger accounts of what people do, think, feel

[4] However, one method can also reveal facets of various criteria. Conversation Analysis, for instance, can illuminate certain aspects of all criteria (Stommel, 2008).

etc. (e.g., Potter and Wetherell, 1987; Widdicombe and Wooffitt, 1995). It appears that in conversation, speakers often display oppositional attitudes depending on the conversational instant.[5] Hence, there is reason not to focus merely on members' attitudes or feelings, but also on their discursive practices. Korenman and Wyatt considered to what extent users follow the forum guidelines and discourse styles (oral vs. written), but did not go deeper into the unfolding interactions of the forum. Being both researchers *and* members of the group, they concluded that their impression that the interaction in the forum felt like interaction within a group can be explained by a high rate of personal email messages in contrast to messages addressing the entire list and a high degree of oral discourse style. Although the relevance of addressing and discourse style is not questioned as such, it remains unclear on which grounds an online group can be labeled a virtual community. It seems that certain practices lead to a "feeling of community," which implies that community is the outcome of certain practices. On the other hand, certain criteria of community are viewed as means or "tools" with which to build a community (e.g., oral-like discourse, frequent participation, etc.). To summarize, studies of online support groups have not taken into account the issue of community, and studies of community in other online groups are caught in a cleavage that divides observable criteria from feelings of community.

Alternative: Online community as an accomplishment

The dilemma between criteria for community and feelings of community is probably relevant not only for research purposes, but also for everyday "community" life, including forums, newsgroups, MUDs, and other online environments. According to Preece (2000), the way members interact contributes to the community's evolution, but, at the same time, its evolution depends on the community's purpose, member roles and policies/rules. These factors help make each online community unique; each one has its own form of community. Therefore, it seems important to analyze how social actors actually deal with *community* in the specific setting of the community as it occurs naturally (i.e., not experimentally). Hence, we need an approach that favors a study of how *members* understand and practice community, in which understandings and practices are not separated but considered as intricately interconnected. This could be offered via a discursive perspective informed by ethnomethodology and conversation analysis (CA).

Ethnomethodology is interested in people's shared methods of making sense in the social world, which is also called *practical reasoning* (Garfinkel,

---

[5] Potter and Wetherell (1987) have demonstrated how people enact oppositional attitudes about emigrants and racism within a single conversation without appearing contradictory or inconsequent.

1967). This means that it treats social life, including "community," as the business that people conduct with each other, displayed in their everyday practices. As a consequence, if we wish to study community from this perspective, it requires a detailed analysis of the actors' *practices* by which they accomplish a community. Another way of putting it is the focus on the participants' "doing" of community. Thus, the dilemma of relying either on the participants' feelings or on the distinct discursive phenomena is relaxed. Community should not be defined a priori, but should be seen as both an "outcome" of and a "rationale" for situated practice.[6] As the central "naturally occurring" practice in an online forum is the exchange of textual messages, the community is accomplished in these chains of contributions (if at all).[7] Since, from an ethnomethodological/conversation analytic stance, it is assumed that the details of the everyday world in mundane conversation are not "an inherently disorderly and unresearchable mess" (Heritage, 2001: 48) but, on the contrary, orderly, then a detailed analysis of interaction is the methodological road to take (see also section 4.5).

However, in online forums, these interactive messages are not uncontrolled, despite their natural occurring status. Structures external to the interaction guide, restrict or sanction participants' actions in a different way than in face-to-face interactions, either mundane or institutional. These include Internet access, "opening hours" of the forum, synchronicity versus asynchronicity of the interaction, the moderators' activity in the forum, but also the forum's Rules and Regulations.[8] Leaving such regulatory structures out of the analytical scope would narrow down the scope of the findings of an interaction analysis. Hence, a concept of community as the product (or outcome) and re-

---

[6] Probably the most revolutionary example of this way of conceptualizing categories of social life is the perspective on gender as "doing" gender, which is understood as: "an emergent feature of social situations: both as an outcome of and a rationale for various social arrangements and as a means of legitimating one of the most fundamental divisions of society" (West and Zimmerman, 1987: 126). With reference to Garfinkel's (1967) study of Agnes, an MTF transsexual who learned to pass for a "normal" and "natural" woman, displaying gender was viewed as a practical task.

[7] The methodical assumption is that of the routine observability of social activities (Francis and Hester, 2004: 23). This implies that the researcher can observe practices just like any member of society, because s/he is equipped with the same kinds of social competences that any member can be assumed to possess.

[8] Naturally, society is also more generally characterized by structures that function as ramifications for individuals' actions (Giddens, 1984). In this view, structures are both the input and output of human actions. These actions in turn have both intended and unintended consequences. Although actors know a great deal about "input" structures, they do not know all about it.

source (or rationale) of interaction requires a certain framework. Goffman's (1974) concept of *frame* is useful in this regard. The *frame* of an activity is the common, practically realized understanding of the meaning and organizational premises of interaction:

> It has been argued that a strip of activity will be perceived by its participants in terms of the rules or premises of a primary framework, whether social or natural .... It has also been argued that these frameworks are not merely a matter of mind but correspond in some sense to the way in which an aspect of the activity itself is organized – especially activity directly involving social agents. Organizational premises are involved, and these are something cognition somehow arrives at, not something cognition creates or generates. Given their understanding of what it is that is going on, individuals fit their actions to this understanding and ordinarily find that the ongoing world supports this fitting. These organizational premises – sustained both in the mind and in activity – I call the frame of the activity (Goffman, 1974: 247).

Taking into account the frame of interactions or practices thus requires a scrutiny of the organizational premises. The organizational premises of online support groups include both aspects of system structure, management and moderation, but also Rules and Regulations or *netiquette*.

Focusing on the influence of online support group Rules and Regulations, it seems that the conceptualization of community as an accomplishment can be supplemented by or combined with an understanding of the status of such rules based on the theory of Community of Practice (Lave and Wenger, 1991; Wenger, 1998). Organizational premises and actual interaction or other discursive practices are theoretically connected in Community of Practice theory. The advantage of this approach is thus that the interconnection between the criteria for community is not dependent on *distinct* approaches, but can also be theoretically explained (Stommel, 2008). Forum rules are put into practice and referred to in the interaction, but they are defined, and thus exist, also external to interaction. Practice and experience with forum interactions may lead to modifications or changes in the rules, while other practices in forum interactions are sanctioned on the basis of these rules. This interrelation between forum rules and (interactive) practices needs to be taken into account when studying online communities. The conceptual framework of Community of Practice (CoP) offers an understanding of how reified rules and statements co-occur with participation in communities, and thus can be used for studying online support groups.[9] I will briefly sketch the relevant aspects of CoP theory in the next section.

---

[9] I intentionally do not coin the merging of virtual community and CoP "virtual community of practice," since this would cause confusion with another use of the term Virtual Communities of Practice (VCoP) as used by Dubé et al. (2006).

1.6 Community of Practice as the *frame* of community accomplishment

A framework that encompasses both external structures and the agency (the "doing") on the side of participants is the concept of Community of Practice (Lave and Wenger, 1991). People form CoPs as they pursue shared enterprises over time, which are always situated in socio-historical, cultural and institutional contexts. The CoP approach destabilizes an essential, permanent and unified understanding of community. Eckert and McConnell-Ginet, who introduced the concept to the fields of sociolinguistics, linguistic anthropology and related disciplines, have defined Community of Practice as

> [a]n aggregate of people who come together around mutual engagement in an endeavor. Ways of doing things, ways of talking, beliefs, values, power relations – in short, practices – emerge in the course of this mutual endeavor. As a social construct, a CofP is different from the traditional community, primarily because it is defined simultaneously by its membership and by the practice in which that membership engages (1992: 464).

In the CoP concept, meaning, identity, practice and community are relational and mutually constitutive. In this spectrum, language use or interaction is covered by the term practice. Community is intricately connected and mutually constitutive with meaning and identity. As Wenger puts it: "[P]articipation in Communities of Practice shapes not only what we do, but also who we are and how we interpret what we do" (Wenger, 2004: 4).

The negotiation of meaning in CoPs involves two constituent processes, namely participation and reification, which must be understood as a duality. The conceptual pair "participation-reification" can explain the relevance of the forum's Rules and Regulations in interactions. Participation (together with reification) describes the social experience of living in the world in terms of membership in social communities and one's active involvement in social enterprises. It is both personal and social. Reification refers to the marks produced by human activity, and refers both to the product and to the process of this marking. Reification and participation, as fundamental to the concept of CoP, are not mutually exclusive, but complementary and always in interplay. The question of whether interaction is a form of participation or a form of reification cannot be answered unambiguously. It is stated that words as projections of human meaning are a form of reification, but that at the same time words in speech "affect the negotiation of meaning through a process that seems like pure participation" (Wenger, 2004: 62). In other words, interaction is the negotiation of meaning and therefore encompasses processes of both reification and participation. Hence, not only documents such as Rules and Regulations are reifications, but verbal interaction itself also has reificative dimensions.

Generally, the reificative dimension in online interaction is stronger than in ephemeral face-to-face conversation. In many web-based forums, interactions are automatically stored in an archive, and are therefore retraceable. As a result, the history of the forum is publicly available. Nonetheless, these reified interactions are results of the negotiation of meaning in time and space by various participants. In many web-based forums, threads stored in the archive can be modified and deleted by participants themselves. Thus, the reified forum interactions remain subjected to participatory activities. Furthermore, the Rules and Regulations have been shaped by the experience of the moderators' participation. Reified in a web-based document, these rules are markers of both the forum's history and culture.

In CoP, community is closely linked to identity. The bridge between the two is membership, through which identities are constructed: "Building an identity consists of negotiating the meanings of our experience of membership in social communities" (Wenger, 2004: 145). In other words, membership serves as the pivot between the social and the individual. Furthermore, membership is seen as something internally constructed in the community. Group boundaries are maintained but not necessarily defined in contrast with outgroups. Rather, membership in a community translates into an "identity as a form of competence" (Wenger, 2004: 153). With this idea, Lave and Wenger (1991) positioned themselves against a conceptualization of learning as internalization. They criticized the notion that a sharp dichotomy between "inside" and "outside" presumes an unproblematic view on the individual as a unit of analysis and moreover, learning is too easily seen as "absorbing the given." In contrast to learning as internalization, they proposed learning as an increased level of participation in CoPs. Thus, learning is considered the engagement in practice through which new members move from the community's periphery to its core. This implies that membership boundaries are permeable; today's peripheral members can be a community's core members tomorrow. As the key to legitimate peripheral participation, newcomers do not learn *from* talk (instruction), but they learn *to* talk.

Some exemplary moments or aspects in which the influence of organizational/technical premises or "things" external to the interaction in an online support group is undeniable are the duality of reification and participation and the issue of membership. As was mentioned above, an analysis of online interaction must somehow take into account the online support group's Rules and Regulations as reifications. Whether participants really (consciously or unconsciously) take into account rules concerning language ("Do not describe things in this or that manner") or behavior ("Be friendly, respectful, constructive etc.") remains questionable, but forum moderators who delete words or descriptions from members' postings do this with explicit reference to the forum rules. Thus, the rules obviously interfere with one's participation. However, participation also influences reification when the forum rules are adapted on the basis of increased experience gathered through participative practice.

Nicknames are another example of reifications closely linked to participation. Members choose their own nickname, but as they send off the chosen name, they may receive an automatic reply saying that the chosen nickname already exists in the forum. Participants may also register again under a different nickname (for whatever reason). Still, the reificative aspect of nicknames is rather strong, since changing a nickname is impossible or forbidden in most online forums because it obstructs the recognizability of members.
Furthermore, peripheral members of CoPs develop their membership through participation, in other words, through "doing" being a member. This implies that the community facilitates multiple (potentially hierarchically organized) fashions of engaging in a practice, which somehow display membership. From an ethnomethodological, or conversation analytical perspective, membership practices are "oriented to" in the actual conduct of the interaction. Both CoP and ethnomethodology/CA thus deny the existence of fixed membership roles. This enables increased sensitivity towards the fact that a group can be reluctant to accept a newcomer, despite the fact that s/he has registered and composed a first posting and is thus already factually present as a novice member. As mentioned above, Galegher et al. (1998) have suggested that a reason for being ignored could be a lack of demonstrated legitimacy. Compare a patient who has been assigned to a particular therapy group (Sacks, 1992): Through (interactional) behavior, other members of the group point out that membership is something that needs to be developed, for instance, by inviting or not inviting a newcomer into a room. As Sacks noted: "Management can bring him in, i.e., say 'Come in', but can't make him a member of the group, i.e., say 'Join in'" (1992: 319). In this situation, the issue of an invitation may be concerned with whatever challenge the group is going to make against the management represented by the therapist. But it also means that novice members, presumably aspiring to being accepted, may do something to gain an invitation.

These preliminary considerations mean that CoP offers a concept of community that is combinable with the understanding of online community as an accomplishment. It does not rely on community feelings, nor on distinct criteria, but allows a theoretical linking of participation with factors, such as Rules and Regulations, nicknames and membership.

1.7 Conclusion

Previous research on online support groups suggested that they are beneficial for healing and some studies suggested that this success (in part) depends on social issues that seem related to community aspects, such as one's legitimacy to become a member. Thus far, the relevance of being a community has not been analyzed for online support groups. The present study will analyze these social aspects of online support groups. This research aim, however, requires a definition of community. Definitions of community found in previous research on online or virtual communities seem to rely on feelings of community versus observable criteria that could indicate the "degree" of community. Alternatively, I propose an ethnomethodological/interactional approach, which sees community as an accomplishment. I am also aware, however, that an empirical study of community as an (interactional) accomplishment should be attentive to issues that are not directly observable in the actual interaction, but are important aspects of the "frame" of the interaction, such as reification (for example, Rules and Regulations and nicknames) and membership. I argue that CoP can serve as a frame for a concept of community as the accomplishment of the participants in a naturally occurring online setting, as it understands interaction as practice (being primarily participatory but also reificatory) related to membership (as a pivot between identity and community and not fixed). Thus, I generally avoid arguing that CoP and ethnomethodology/CA are theoretically reconcilable approaches: For such a statement the relation between the two would have to be investigated in depth [Stommel, 2008]). For the present study, the frame in which the community is accomplished is not the subject of investigation itself, although the awareness that there is such a frame is repeatedly touched upon. Since "doing" community and membership are in interplay with identity, the following chapter develops an approach to identity that complements the ethnomethodological/CA perspective on community I will take.

Chapter 2

Identity in a community

2.1 Introduction

One of the questions this study deals with is to what extent it matters "who you are," in the joining process of an online support group. What is identity's role in a community? And what theories and concepts of identity are compatible with the chosen approach to community as something members accomplish in a discursive setting like an online forum?

Identity has been approached in a myriad of ways in various disciplines covering a substantial body of theory from Erikson (1968) to Hall (2004). These approaches can roughly be divided into two competing impulses (cf. Tracy, 2002). On the one hand, identity refers to the stable features of the people involved, and on the other hand, identity is a dynamic and situated accomplishment. The stable features of people are said to exist prior to any particular situation. In contrast, according to the second impulse (engendered by the Linguistic Turn in the social sciences), identity changes from one occasion to the next, corresponding to the idea that it is fragmented and always in flux. For the present research, the focus lies on the dynamic concept of identity, although the possibility of more durable and thus provisionally stable identities is also taken into account.

Section 2.2 sets out to explore the relation between community and identity. Then, in section 2.3, Goffman's theories about identity are proposed as support for the concept of identity as an accomplishment in human interaction. His theory of stigma takes account of "special" rules for identity for those in society with a stigma, among whom ill persons (2.4); hence, accomplishing identity is not the same for each individual. Section 2.5 relates identity accomplishment to poststructuralist considerations of identity and discourses, followed by section 2.6, in which an empirical take on identity accomplishment is adopted from interaction analysts. This focus is well worded by Benwell and Stokoe:

> [A commitment to an empirical and discourse-based understanding of identity] enables us to put some 'flesh' on the bones of an abstract, theorised notion of 'identity', in ways that are empirically rich, methodologically grounded and compatible with some of the most exciting critical theoretical ideas to emerge at the turn of the twenty-first century (2006: 47).

Therefore, the present study takes the approach that identity accomplishment should be studied to comprehend the exact details in which members of an online support group "do" identity in their interactions with others. In section 2.7, three ethnomethodologically informed concepts of identity are distinguished for the actual analysis of an online support group: Categorical identity, situational identity and personal identity.

2.2 The relevance of identity in a community

The fact that the online support groups can have a positive effect has already been mentioned. This may be related to the fact that such groups accommodate the shift from a certain "ill" identity to a healthier one. A change of identity in this sense is thus accommodated by the group or the community in which the individual is situated. This has been considered the success formula of A.A. (Alcoholics Anonymous) (Lave and Wenger, 1991). The explicit goal here is that participants perceive themselves as alcoholics. Newcomers learn this by rehearsing their life stories with close coaching by "old-timers." The purpose of this is not only that they learn the local practice, but that they also learn to see themselves in their situation as fitting into a broader community. As such, belonging to a large community of recovering alcoholics is expected to give them the courage to align themselves with the organization and to stay sober. Lave and Wenger explained:

> In A.A. … discussions have a dual purpose. Participants engage in the work of staying sober and they do so through gradual construction of an identity. Telling the personal story is a tool of diagnosis and reinterpretation. Its communal use is essential to the fashioning of an identity as a recovered alcoholic, and thus to remaining sober. It becomes a display of membership by virtue of fulfilling a crucial function in the shared practice (1991: 109).

This implies that identity operates at various levels in the community's practices. The individual is motivated by a socially (including juridically or medically) defined stigma (alcoholic, mentally ill, criminal) to enter the community, and is ascribed the community-based identity "newcomer." Through the processes of learning and engagement (which involves some initiation in the beginning), this community identity develops towards an identity of a recovered alcoholic together with the process of becoming a regular or experienced member. The very beginning of the participation process in the community is crucial, not only because the community members treat the novice in a certain way, but also because the step involving joining embodies the commencement of a change. A medical professional has formulated this type of change in the area of pathological gambling and the activities of Gambling Anonymous:

> Consider the anonymous movements. One of the great rituals that is performed there is that a person introduces themselves [*sic*] and engages in a deliberately self-stigmatizing act: Hi, I'm Joe and I'm an alcoholic... or addict... or compulsive gambler... or whatever. I would argue that when a person advances that public statement about themselves [*sic*], they [*sic*] at once profess and reconstruct who they [*sic*] are. This event is an act of positive stigma – the person asserts that this is an important distinction about who they [*sic*] are, and more importantly what they [*sic*] are trying to do about it. So, the person is paradoxically more and less a gambler/addict/whatever when they [*sic*] come to this point. They [*sic*] are taking up the mantle of the stigmatic identity and at the same time leaving it behind and taking up the ethic of abstinence (Grunfeld et al., 2004: 8).

In other words, admitting that you are addicted is considered the first step in the healing process. This observation points in the direction of the crucial role of discourse regarding identity. Putting things into words in a specific context may actually effect a change.

The relevance of identity in a community does not lie solely in the hands of the newcomer, who is able to (verbally) accomplish certain identities. Other members also play a crucial role, which is exemplified by observations of the process of admission of new "members" in *total institutions* such as prisons, concentration camps and mental hospitals (Goffman, 1961).[10] Total institutions can be circumscribed as "forcing houses for changing persons; each is a natural experiment on what can be done to the self" (Goffman, 1961: 12). Hence, as in the case of A.A., the community is designed to allow members to achieve a change of the self. This coercion starts with the admission process when an inmate or patient first enters an institution. The novice entering an institution is first stripped of the social arrangements of his old life (clothes, possessions, haircut, etc.). An initial moment of socialization may involve an obedience test, which can be both fostered by the staff or other inmates. One could metaphorically call the initiation a "welcome" or a "rite of passage" (Goffman, 1961: 18). Moreover, the novice experiences role dispossession. The role s/he has previously played in the "real" world (such as a profession) does not play a role in the institution. Even the novice's name may be taken away and replaced by a form of address used by inmates. All in

[10] Foucault (1967, 1977) also analyzed several types of total institutions, but these are less of interest for the present study, because he traced historical changes (rather than contemporary settings) and analyzed texts as products of discourses, rather than the actual conduct of interactional practices.

all, the territories of the self (both bodily and symbolically, i.e., through humiliation) are violated. The mortification of identity in the total institution is therefore assumed to cause considerable stress for the novice. The diffuse and strictly enforced regulations may be expected to cause the novice to live with chronic anxiety about breaking the rules and the consequence of breaking them (Goffman, 1961: 42). In fact, to avoid possible incidents, the novice may forego certain levels of sociability with his fellow inmates or patients.

Online support groups are, of course, barely comparable with total institutions. However, Goffman's observations and those regarding groups like A.A. offer some indications of what an analysis of online support groups should be sensitive to. Identity seems particularly relevant at the moment a novice member enters the community, and may be articulated by some form of welcoming ritual. The change of the self, which is frequently strived for by the group or the institution, seems to be facilitated by the social situation of being in a group, which suggests the relevance of the community. The emphasis on identity change is not to suggest that the present study could actually document or measure such changes in individual cases. This would involve an investigation of the formation of the self, or personal identity, which goes beyond the emphasis on identity and community in a specific process in online support groups. However, it does indicate the potential relevance of identity (including how you present yourself and how you are being treated) in online support groups in relation to the status of the group as a community.

2.3 Identity as a social, performative and interactional accomplishment

This chapter develops a concept of identity that serves the analysis of the interconnection between community and identity, more specifically illness as an identity. Because mental illness does not change from one moment to the next, it is commonsensically viewed as a more or less durable characteristic of an individual. Nevertheless, in a specific social situation, such as entering a group, it requires some form of enactment, or accomplishment by the ill individual. This section argues for an understanding of illness as a social identity, which implicates a non-cognitive, situational perspective on social identity. Whereas Social Identity Theory seems inappropriate in this context for reasons I will go into, Goffman's theory of identity is more useful.

Social Identity Theory: cognitive and pre-discursive

Because community is approached through the Community of Practice *frame*, identity or the self is seen in close relation to community. This means that the interest of the present study is primarily involved with an understanding of the self as social and intersubjective. When we view the individual as socially located, the self is defined by virtue of its membership of, or identification with a particular group. One way of theorizing this social character is to speak of collective or group identities, which include gender, race, class, etc. The most well-known approach in this field is probably Social Identity Theory (SIT) and the related Social Categorisation Theory (SCT), developed by Tajfel and Turner (e.g., Tajfel, 1982; Tajfel and Turner, 1986). In these theories, social identity is opposed to personal identity, and refers to the individual's identification with a group, which includes a certain reflexivity regarding group membership and the emotional attachment or specific disposition of belonging to the group. SIT examines "in-group" and "out-group" processes of membership, which means that, depending on the activity an individual is engaged in, s/he constitutes the "in-group" to which s/he belongs, and the "out-group" to which s/he does not belong. This is a cognitive process that serves particular social and psychological goals, such as boosting one's self-esteem. Thus, social identity, or rather group membership, is seen as something to be switched on by the individual depending on the social situation. For this, SIT has been fundamentally criticized (e.g., Widdicombe and Wooffitt, 1995). It assumes that identity is a cognitive and pre-discursive phenomenon and thus fails to offer a truly social understanding of it, which is connected to the concept of identity as an accomplishment.

Goffman's social, performative, interactional concept of identity

In contrast to the cognitive grounds of SIT, Goffman's (1959) perspective on identity is intricately tied to the social, and more specifically, the dramaturgical. The concepts of *performance*, *facework/impression management* and *rituals* together constitute this social, but moreover interactional, approach to identity. The mundane world is considered a stage with actors and an audience and interaction is the performance that takes place on the stage. Performances allow individuals to present themselves and their activities in everyday life as an attempt to guide and control the impressions others have of them. The performance exists regardless of the mental state of the individual, because identity attributes or social roles (also called *persona*) are often imputed to the individual in spite of her/his lack of faith in – or even ignorance of – this performance. Goffman (1959: 18) used the example of the doctor who decides to give a placebo to a patient, fully aware of its impotence, because of the patient's desire for more extensive treatment. In this way, the individual develops identity or persona as a function of interaction with others, through an exchange of information.

Goffman's (1967) concept of *facework* is another important aspect in the understanding of identity in human interaction. It refers to the rules for face-to-face social interaction (also referred to by the term *impression management*). When face is maintained, it engenders a positive feeling. Put differently:

> Each individual ... presents a self that he or she considers desirable, and that he or she figures others will be willing to acknowledge and support in the interaction. ... Face, then, can be seen as the social glue that keeps people attuned to each other in interaction – it is what keeps them coordinating their actions closely (Eckert and McConnell-Ginet, 2003: 59).

Disruptions of this, or losing face, result in a loss of the internal emotional support that is protecting oneself in a social situation. In order to save face, one must be socially perceptive. Face saving is not just a process of the social actor, but of the audience as well. There are social protocols for helping someone maintain and save face, most notably avoidance mechanisms, overcompensating and apology. More specifically, there is a ritual around correcting the way in which face is managed socially – challenge, offering, acceptance and thanks (Goffman, 1967: 22). According to Goffman (1982/1971), rituals can be described as conventionally organized bundles of performances. He defines ritual practices as mechanical, conventionalized actions, found not only in primitive cultures, but also in urbanized, mundane settings (Goffman, 1982: 139). They are dialogical in the sense that if one person politely offers another individual something, the other is expected to act reciprocally in a polite fashion by, for instance, displaying gratefulness. These two actions – offering and thanking – constitute a small ceremony, which is an affirmative exchange. When the rules of the ceremony are broken, a corrective exchange must take place to heal the social relationship of the parties. According to Goffman, affirmative and corrective exchanges are the most frequent rituals, or conventionalized and mechanically conducted actions, performed in human interaction. Goffman's ideas sustain the view of identity as an accomplishment, and make it clear that identity is not a goal in itself but a function of human interaction. His perspective on stigma explains that the rules for human interaction depend on the participants' stigmatized attributes.

2.4 Differentiating identities: Stigma

The focus on impression management ignores the more permanent characteristics of the actual interactants, which are perceivable to or known by the co-interactants. They are rather general descriptions of social interaction, excluding that social relationships may be influenced by the fact that one interactant is socially different. A concept that takes into account the possibility of being different is *stigma* (Goffman, 1986). Stigma can be circumscribed as a deeply discrediting attribute that invokes shame and uneasiness in a particular situation. A stigma can be a physical trait or a "blemish of individual character" (Goffman, 1986: 4), which may mean mental disorder, addiction, suicide attempts, physical handicaps, etc. However, the same attribute may be a stigma in one context and not in another. A stigma is thus a special kind of *relationship* between attribute and stereotype. People anticipate certain categories and attributes in encountering another individual. When a deeply discrediting attribute disrupts the normative expectations that one may have about someone else,[11] this attribute is a stigma.

Stigma works in two directions. On the one hand, there are *discredited* attributes that are either already known or immediately evident. On the other hand, when the individual assumes the attribute is neither known nor perceivable by those present, the attribute is still *discreditable* and the individual will try to hide it. Impression management, which is something all social actors do, is even more obvious with stigmatized individuals. Those who are discredited must deal with the tension their stigma causes in order to successfully interact with others, while those suffering from a "hidden" stigma are forced to try to limit access to information about that stigma.

In a particular phase of the socialization process, the stigmatized person learns and incorporates the wider societal beliefs about the stigma and what it is like to have it. An inborn stigma must be clearly distinguished from the socialization pattern of the one who becomes (or becomes aware of) it later in life. When someone falls ill with a severe (life-threatening or chronic) disease, the individual not only has to deal with the disease itself, but also with the social stigma as something that demands the individual to assume a new role. It has even been claimed that illness requires the acquisition of a new identity: "Sickness is an identity that must be assumed, acquired and imposed on others" (Herzlich and Pierret, 1985: 147). The emphasis on idealized, normative identity and conduct limits the ability of the discredited individual to achieve full acceptance by the population that s/he is forced to assimilate into. For the potentially discredited individual who attempts to "pass" and employ "disidentifiers" to establish her/himself as "normal" (Goffman, 1986: 44), feelings of ambivalence and alienation emerge as a result of one's limited social intercourse. These may translate into motives to join a local, stigmatized community in which one can be "oneself."

In Goffman's view of stigma and face-to-face encounters, the stigmatized person's way of dealing with the stigma in relation to society at large was at the center of attention. When Goffman spoke of communities or groups of stigmatized people, it was in terms of politics in the broadest sense of the term and not in terms of their internal communication. However, he specifi-

[11] Goffman (1986:2-3) described this as the discrepancy between virtual social identity and actual social identity.

cally noticed how common group formation amongst stigmatized individuals is:

> [T]here are the huddle-together self-help clubs formed by the divorced, the aged, the obese, the physically handicapped, the ileostomied and colostomied. There are residential clubs, voluntary to varying degrees, formed for the ex-alcoholic and the ex-addict. There are national associations such as AA which provide a full doctrine and almost a way of life for their members (Goffman, 1986: 22).

What a stigmatized identity means or what role it plays in an actual community and how this community works was not investigated by Goffman. It could be that in a community of stigmatized individuals, the norms of impression management concerning the stigma are different than from general society's hegemonic social norms. Hence, whereas Goffman explored the characteristics of the stigmatized with relation to normal people, the present study focuses instead on a potential relevance of stigma in encounters of members of a stigma-community.

Relying on the understanding of identity offered by Goffman's work means that identities are carried out in human interaction, and thus are also expressed in language. However, Goffman's approach suggests that the individual consciously manages the impressions s/he makes. The subject is thereby ascribed a far-reaching consciousness and powerful role in directing other people's impressions of her/him.[12] The concept of stigma means that dealing with illness as an identity implies societal norms and expectations, which cannot be managed freely. This lack of a subject's agency is well-explained by poststructuralist theory, which describes that identities are embedded in and invoked by discourses. I will briefly situate the approach of identity as an accomplishment in a discursive context.

2.5 Identity embedded in discourses

From a poststructuralist point of view, identity is a (social) construction, a process that is never completed (Hall, 2004). This means that identity is non-essentialist, multiple and variable, and implies that an individual does not have one or more true identities. Gender, occupation, sexuality, nationality,

---

[12] Another point of critique is that Goffman's analyses are merely descriptive generalizations of stigma and total institutions and thus he presents neither an account for alternative forms of conduct with regard to stigmatized identity nor the fine details of identity construction.

religion, etc. are social categories that can potentially be activated as relevant identities. Poststructuralists see the political need to exploit a notion of identities in discourses, whilst acknowledging that these are temporary attachments, and not essentially "cores" of self. Ideology and hegemonic practices operate to impose stability and fixation upon the shifts of signifiers in the discursive field, which renders subjects "gendered," "sexualized" or "racialized."

According to Foucault (1972), dominant discourses, tied to social arrangements and practices, discursively produce the subject. Butler has analyzed the discursive production of the gendered subject and concluded: "[T]here is no gender identity behind the expressions of gender; that identity is performatively constituted by the very 'expressions' that are said to be its results" (1990: 33). Thus, identity is a performance and a discursive practice, implying non-essentialism and transience. This means that Butler applied the term performance, although she denied that the performing subject relies on an agentive and rational self to manage impressions or facework (as Goffman did, see above).

Naturally, the one-to-one internalization of discourses is an inadequate explanation of the formation of the subject. Rather, psychoanalytical ideas of identification must be adopted to explain that the subject is not merely "interpellated" in a purely passive sense, but reflexively recognizes and invests in this position. The power of discourse in producing subjectivities is assumed, but the subject is also able to bring forth change. According to Butler, a discursive concept of identity essentially contains this paradox: "Subjection consists precisely in this fundamental dependency on a discourse we never choose but that, paradoxically, initiates and sustains our agency" (1997: 2). Subversion or disruption of these discourses can occur through performances (Butler, 1990). On the one hand, the endless repetition of performances constructs seemingly fixed subjectivities or identities, but, on the other hand, this repetition allows for, even guarantees, the possibility of change, since the repetition is never completely identical with its original. Thus, each new performance entails the possible disruption of the structure through *resignification*. In this manner, a discursive approach to identity can account for both structure and agency.

To summarize, poststructuralist discursive approaches "describe identity as a fluid, dynamic and shifting process, capable of both reproducing and destabilising the discursive order" (Benwell and Stokoe, 2006: 34). It is, however, an approach, which does not pay attention to how people in their everyday lives do these performances in interaction with others. Other discourse approaches that employ an ethnomethodological approach, such as conversation analysis, shy away from an abstract theoretization of discourse as a producer of subjects to "the analytic exemplification of discourse as a social practice" (Speer and Potter, 2002: 152). The present study sets out to investigate the actual accomplishment of identity, whilst it acknowledges the more structural interconnection of identities with discourses.

2.6 The actual "doing" of identity in interaction

The so-called grand theories of identity (i.e., poststructuralist theory) usually do not answer the question of how identities are discursively constructed or performed in practice or in "real" life. Ethnomethodologists and conversation analysts prefer to approach identity accomplishment (or identity construction, or performance) from an empirical, analytical perspective, rather than a theoretical one. A few assumptions are relevant in this regard. Ethnomethodologists are interested in mundane settings in which identities are enacted, preferably in face-to-face interaction, rather than in written text. Furthermore, it is assumed that this interaction is contingent, but not disorderly. This warrants the ethnomethodological project of explicating members' methods to help produce orderly and accountable social activities (Garfinkel, 1967). These activities mostly occur in language or, as CA calls it, in *talk-in-interaction*. According to Schegloff (1992), this is the primordial site of human sociality. It is through talking that we live our lives, build and maintain relationships and establish "who we are to one another" (Drew, 2005, cit. in Benwell and Stokoe, 2006: 36). This is not to say that material, or corporeal aspects do not influence identity, but to instead focus on how these "real" things are dealt with in how people communicate with one another in a variety of settings and/or communities. From this point of view, identity is seen as "doing" identity *in interaction*.

In interaction, multiple and variable identities can be performed and achieved, but also resisted (and thus, the poststructuralist's emphasis on the variable and multiple understanding of identities is accounted for). This presupposes that identities as group categories (including stigma categories such as prisoner, blind person or someone with an eating disorder) are resources for individuals that can be both resisted and adopted in interaction with others. The local context of the talk is crucial for the employment of such categories. Two examples of Widdicombe and Wooffitt's (1995) study of subcultural identities (e.g., rockers, Goths, punks, etc.) are illustrative of this point. The researchers conducted informal interviews with people on the street and at music festivals. Consider the beginning of one of their interviews with two female punks, presented as excerpt 1.

Excerpt 1[13]

(Tape starts)

1	I:	about your sty:le
2		(.3)
3	I:	and who you are
4		(.4)
5		how would you describe yourselves
6	R1:	huhh huhh hhagh punk rockers
7	R2:	punk rockers yeah huhh huhh
8	I:	How long have you been punk rockers,
9	R2:	three:- ah've been three years
10	R1:	yeah three

Source: Widdicombe and Wooffitt (1995: 81).

The turn-by-turn organization of talk as a convention makes the respondents' answers in line 6 and 7 sequentially relevant and the fact that these respondents stick to this convention displays their tacit knowledge of it. According to Widdicombe and Wooffitt, these interviewees not only have tacit knowledge of the turntaking organization of interaction, but also of the type of exchange that is taking place between them and two interviewers they have never met before. The researchers reported that many respondents, prior to the interview proper, spontaneously remarked that they had never been interviewed before. This confirms the notion that they had a label, or a definition of the situation – the interview. In other words, these people know they are being interviewed, and basic tacit knowledge informs the respondents' interpretation of the interviewer's first utterance. One of the features of interviews is that the interviewer elicits the "enactment" of an identity by the interviewee right at the beginning. The respondents must make sense of the fact that *they* were picked out for this interview by the researchers. In the case of this study on subcultures the interviewers selected individuals that looked strikingly different to other people in the street at the time. In this way, the tacit basic knowledge of the situation – the interview – and the specific situation of looking different than other people in the street, made the subcultural category relevant as a response to the question in line 5.

In other words, the situation, an interview (but also an online support group) makes certain actions more appropriate than others. This does not mean, however, that the respondent is in any way committed to producing that action. Sequences of actions are not deterministic because not producing the action is also a communicative resource. The category punk rocker in excerpt

[13] See Widdicombe and Wooffitt (1995) for the explanation of their transcription symbols.

1 above is argued to be sequentially relevant. Consequentially, *not* declaring yourself incumbent of a category where it is sequentially relevant is a form of resistance. Consider excerpt 2.

Excerpt 2

(Tape starts)

1	I:	how would you descry:be (.) yourself
2		and appearance and so on
3		(.)
4	R:	describe my appearance
5	I:	yeah
6		(1)
7	R:	su-su-slightly longer than average hair
		(Respondent goes on to provide an account of his appearance)

Source: Widdicombe and Wooffitt (1995: 86).

Widdicombe and Wooffitt analyzed this exchange as saliently *not* delivering a self-categorization in terms of group membership. This does not mean that the interviewee does not see himself as a rocker, but rather that at this very moment of the conversation (the very beginning) he resists the employment of a subcultural identity. When the interviewee is asked a few lines later whether he would call himself a rocker, he says yes, which implies that articulating a certain social identity is closely bound to the local context of the conversation. This cannot be explained by a cognitive approach, since the social context (in terms of in-group vs. out-group) has not changed. Therefore, Widdicombe and Wooffitt (1995: 109) have proposed approaching identity more empirically, rather than theoretically, in order to appreciate how different identities are achieved and resisted in turn-by-turn sequences of talk, and the local functions that are served.

This implies that the following three principles of identity in a conversation are central to the analysis of identity accomplishment (Antaki and Widdicombe, 1998):

1. Having an identity is being cast into a category with associated features.
2. This casting is indexical and occasioned.
3. Identity is made relevant to, and consequential for, the interactional business at hand, and relies on conversational structures.

Point 1 refers to the observation that identity accomplishment is related to the work of categories in social interaction. I will present more about this in the next section. Point 2 refers to the meaning of identity depending on the local (interactional) setting of occurrence. All language use, or talk-in-context is indexical in the sense that the relevant category to describe a person does not depend on who the person is, but on the occasion of its production. The third point links identity accomplishment to the rules of conversation, such as turn-taking and adjacency pairs (see also section 4.5).

2.7 Three types of identity as an accomplishment

It was mentioned above (1.2.2) that different types of identity could play a role in communities, for instance, the identity of a newcomer simultaneously with an addict. Although both can be seen as accomplishments in interaction, it seems useful to distinguish between the various types.

A. Categorical identities

A commonsense understanding of identity at the very least includes identity in terms of categories, such as man, hairdresser, schizophrenic, white and middle-class. Looking at these from both an ethnomethodological and post-structuralist point of view avoids the presumption that there is an explanatory link between the ontological status of the person and the identity s/he performs. Rather, the focus is on how actors attend to and are attended to by these categories in their daily interactions. Categories have certain features that are "known" by members of a particular culture or society if we can presume that this commonsense knowledge is validated by the fact that people are generally able to communicate and to understand each other's actions. Categories, including identity categories, are organized in collections (Schegloff, 2007). Woman and man belong to the collection gender, hairdresser and researcher to the collection profession, etc. Single categories can belong to various collections and it depends on the setting in which the categories are employed, which collection is appealed. For instance, whether the category "baby" is a member of the collection family members or lovers depends on the context in which it is used (Sacks, 1992). Moreover, categories and members of categories are linked to particular actions, which are called category-bound activities. By mentioning an activity that is category bound, the relevance of the category can be introduced in the scene (for instance, in an online support group on eating disorders, the description of a binge makes the category bulimia with binging as a typical feature relevant. Another aspect is that categories are viewed as inference rich, which means that the knowledge that ordinary people have about what people are like, how they behave, etc., is referred to and accessed by various *categories of person*, such as student or professor, Muslim or Catholic.

What is crucial for an ethnomethodological approach, as already noted, is a focus on speakers' or actors' categories, which may be categories that the researcher is unaware of beforehand. For instance, the term "hotrodder" was used by teenagers in a group therapy session in the 1960s; Sacks (1992) analyzed how participants used this term to signal membership of the category. Since the therapist used the word "teenagers" to describe the same people, it was pointed out that the term "hotrodder" was essentially a category used by the members themselves. For this reason, Sacks stressed its potential for social change and claimed the term to be a "revolutionary category."

Gender can also be viewed as a members' category, which can be accomplished in online support groups by using nicknames. Names are traditionally either male or female. Of all the information that names can communicate, gender is the most common (Alford, 1988). Even if we do not know anything about a person apart from the first name, we are usually able to categorize that person as female or male, and consequently address her/him in the appropriate manner: *Ms*. or *Mr*., *she* or *he* (Oelkers, 2004). Research on chat conversation has suggested that this is partly true for Internet nicknames as well (Panyametheekul and Herring, 2003; Zelenkauskaite and Herring, 2006). The studies on gender and chat communication reveal that researchers often determine a participant's gender based on their nicknames, although Panyametheekul and Herring (2003) also found "gender indeterminate" nicknames. This suggests that the choice or construction of a nickname is likely to, but must not, establish gender. A focus on gender as one aspect of identity implies that names can ascribe identity attributes of an extremely strict kind. An infant, in its first days of life, shifts from "it," to "she" or "he," essentially by being given a girl's or a boy's name (Butler, 1993). This naming activity shows how a human being is brought into language and kinship through the gendered matrix (Butler, 1990). Because of the absence of visible bodily cues of gender and other physical identity markers in textual online environments, nicknames have been conceptualized as "a kind of substitute for the face and the body" (Subrahmanyam et al., 2004: 660). Alternatively, from a poststructuralist point of view, nicknames are arguably not substitutes for the face and the body, but, rather, constitutive of the self (cf. Butler, 1993).

B. Situational identities

The concept of *situational identity* has been proposed by Zimmerman (1998) in his analysis of emergency calls. Situational identities come into play in particular situations; in the case of emergency calls, the situation can be described as one in which the identities "citizen" and "complainant" are relevant. This is significant for an empirical analysis, since certain expectations are tied to these identities. For instance, the citizen is expected to describe some kind of emergency (more or less) adequately. When s/he fails to realize the category-bound feature of being a citizen-caller, it may have consequences for the subsequent exchange.

In specific settings such as mental hospitals or online forums, the situation also makes the identity of "new patient" or "help-seeker" relevant.

These are clearly related to categorical identities such as "mentally ill" or "sufferer of breast cancer," but how these interconnections are designed remains an empirical question.

C. Personal identities

Apart from the categorical and situational identities observed in discursive practices, identity is also articulated in terms of personality traits or attitudes. These are labeled personal identities (or personal traits), which may include honesty, reasonableness, insecurity, consideration, etc. (Tracy, 2002). Although, like categorical and situational identities, these personal identities are oriented to and accomplished in the course of an interaction, in web-based forums, they are also significantly occasioned by nicknames. Agha's (2007) theory of language and social relations allows for an understanding of nicknames that are textualized in a specific online setting as *indexical demeanors*, which construe the attributes of a particular actor who "wears" a name, partly through the application of stereotypes. In other words, reading nicknames as if one were reading people is a semiotic practice, which is shaped by the (discursive) context, but also by stereotypic social images. Stereotypic images are understood as images associated with signs that specify default ways of reading the people who display them. These stereotypes permit a decontextualized form of circulation, which means that they convert contingent and dialectical facts of persona display into seemingly stable categories of personhood. However, Agha emphasized the significance of the discursive (or textual) context by stating that:

> The indices themselves only become relevant to social interaction under conditions of textuality or co-occurrence with other signs, conditions under which text-level indexical effects superimpose a further specificity upon the current construal, partly canceling, deforming, even troping upon stereotypic effects (2007: 239).

The transfer from stereotypes to the attributes of personhood is achieved by Goffman's concept of *demeanor* (Goffman, 1956). Demeanor can explain how utterances allow interactants to construe attributes, or the personal identity of the speaker. Demeanor is an indexical notion, in the sense that it highlights the connection between attributes displayed by acts and the actor who displays them. The perceivable feature of conduct that contextually conveys the attributes is the demeanor indexical; it clarifies the demeanor of the one who performs the sign. Demeanor indexicals vary with regard to their durability. Some perceivable features of individuals, such as gestures and utterances, are evanescent, while others are seen as more constant characteristics. Distinguishing which characteristics are considered stable and which are less stable requires culture-specific theories of personhood, although, in occidental cultures, psychological and sociological attributions are generally considered temporally constant. It must be stressed, however, that ideas about durability of attributes, ascribed to individuals only by virtue of personal identity indexicals, differ substantially from culture to culture in the degree to which they are objectified as stable, essential, fundamental, and so forth. For online nicknames, however, it may be argued that they perform personal identities of a stable and durable kind, since textually they appear automatically and thus repeatedly with any contribution posted by the actor. In fact, they are instances of reified features of the community, and though they are still subject to participation and thus change, nicknames are difficult or even impossible to change for the participants of an online support group.

2.8 Conclusion

The role of identity upon entering an online community is approached ethnomethodologically, which implies a focus on how members demonstrate who they are to one another and make sense of who others are in the conduct of actual encounters. For online support groups, we need to take into account the potential relevance of stigmas in identity work. A stigma is a highly problematic personal attribute and presumably has to be dealt with in a community devoted to that shared stigma. Identity is theoretically understood as intricately dependent upon discursive practices, as poststructuralists have described, but the focus of this study is more on the investigation of identity in an empirically approachable situation than on the perpetuation of a theoretical explanation of identity. The next chapter considers the aspects of identity, stigma and online support groups with regard to a concrete set of problems, namely eating disorders.

Chapter 3

Accomplishing identity in an online community on eating disorders

3.1 Introduction

Online support groups are regularly launched for all kinds of diseases, syndromes and other problems, including eating disorders. Eating disorders can generally be described as very complex disorders, with an unfavorable prognosis and, in case of anorexia, allegedly the highest mortality rate of all psychic disorders (Gerlinghoff and Backmund, 2004).[14] According to Van Hoeken et al. (2005), both the incidence rate of anorexia (over the past 50 years) and the incidence rate of bulimia (over the 5 years since it was introduced in the DSM III in 1980) have increased. But the statistics on eating disorders are not univocal: The prevalence of anorexia, i.e., the percentage of the female population suffering from anorexia in Germany, has been considered fairly stable,[15] while Westenhöfer (2001) discovered that bulimic behavior decreased in the period 1991 to 1997 in Germany. The prevalence rate among young females lies between 0.5 and 1.5% for anorexia and between 1 and 4% for bulimia in Germany (Gerlinghoff and Backmund, 2004; Herzog et al., 2004; Van Hoeken et al., 2005). The prevalence rate for Binge Eating Disorder (BED) among the German female population lies between 0.7 and 1.5% (Westenhöfer, 2001). Although the debilitating severity of eating disorders in terms of the struggle of those afflicted would be reason enough, the legitimization for conducting a study of an online forum dedicated to eating disorders is more acuminate than that.

In chapter 1, it was suggested that online support groups might be beneficial to those with health-related problems. It was also argued that identities play an important role in various ways in these communities. Chapter 2 proposed the view that (stigmatized) identity was a discursive accomplishment in the ethnomethodological sense of "doing" identity, either through social categories, situational identities or personal identity (in terms of traits or person attributes). Moreover, it was argued that when novice members enter a community, identity is a significant factor for the interaction between the novice and the regulars. The current interest in an online community de-

---

[14] For definitions of the various types of eating disorders, see section 3.2.

[15] According to *AKH-Consilium* (http://www.akh-consilium.at/daten/anorexia.htm).

voted to eating disorders is that novice members will be confronted with certain specific difficulties of eating disorders. Having an eating disorder is not just a fact; there are many facets of eating disorders in social contexts that make it very complicated to "have" one. Although the accountability related to actual eating behavior and bodily appearance in an online forum are "overcome" by the lack of visual cues (Walstrom, 2000b), there is reason to suppose that the mere discussion of the problem on the Internet, or accomplishing the "identity of eating disorders" in an online setting, is potentially entangled with social accountability.

Why should eating disorders be considered "tricky" for novice members of an online forum? This chapter offers three potentially sensitive issues which may play a role here: Gender, eating disorder diagnoses and pro-anorexia. I will elaborate on these issues from a social constructionist perspective, which means that I view eating disorders including their diagnoses, the gender bias and the pro-ana movement as contingent, cultural phenomena.[16] Online communities on eating disorders are players in this sociocultural field. If newcomers join the community, we can expect that they will somehow exhibit or "orient to" the social contingencies of eating disorders. Therefore, this chapter explores which identities that are related to the aspects gender, diagnosis and pro-ana may be relevant for the initiation process involved in joining an online forum. From the proposed ethnomethodological approach, this relevance is not presupposed but considered as tacit background knowledge. Empirically, I examine whether and how participants orient to these various aspects when they become a member of an online support group on eating disorders. The chapter ends with a review of a previous study of an online forum devoted to eating disorders, which indicates the relevance

[16] This view is endorsed by historical and comparative studies. In the first place, a historical change of the aetiology of eating disorders has been observed. The preoccupation with body weight and size (related to the beauty ideal) is a relatively new (20th century) characteristic of eating disorders (Habermas, 1990; Vandereycken et al., 2003). In historical cases of eating disorders, starvation was mainly linked to religious beliefs or social distinction rather than to the preoccupation with weight. In fact, this characteristic (also called "fear of fatness") has only been included in the diagnostic standard DSM IV since 1994 (Gugutzer, 2005). Apart from being historically recent, the fear of fatness in eating disorders has also been argued to be culturally determined, namely associated with westernized and industrialized cultures (Keel and Klump, 2003). It appears that bulimia (with its characteristic purging) is only found in areas of Western influence, and that anorexia's criterion of fear of fatness is a western phenomenon. According to Keel and Klump, anorexia is not culture-bound, if it is limited to the category of self-starvation (i.e., without the fear of fatness). For the current study, the concept of eating disorders is restricted to the contemporary phenomenon of eating disorders related to a westernized lifestyle.

of *being a community* and presenting oneself as eating disordered for an online support group.

3.2 The problem of the medical model: When is a person eating disordered?

In clinical practice, eating disorders are diagnosed on the basis of the international *Diagnostic and Statistical Manual of Mental Disorders,* fourth edition (more commonly referred to as DSM-IV) and the *International Statistical Classification of Diseases and Related Health Problems*, 10th ed. (ICD 10). Combining these two standards, three major types of eating disorders must be distinguished, which can be characterized by the following diagnostic criteria:

Anorexia Nervosa[17]

1. Extreme fear of "fatness."
2. Low body weight/refusal to maintain normal body weight (at least 15% below that expected).
3. The weight loss is self-induced by avoiding "fattening foods" and one or more of the following: Self-induced vomiting; self-induced purging; excessive exercise; use of appetite suppressants and/or diuretics.
4. Loss of menstrual periods in females at least 3 consecutive missed periods. (Additionally, most female sufferers have lost their sexual interest in males.)
5. Distorted body image.

[17] DSM-IV defines two subtypes of anorexia nervosa: (1) a restricting type which is characterized by strict dieting and exercise but without binge eating, (2) a binge-eating and purging type, marked by episodes of compulsive eating with or without self-induced vomiting and the use of laxatives or enemas.

Bulimia Nervosa[18]

1. Extreme fear of "fatness."
2. Preoccupation with eating, and an irresistible craving for food leading to episodes of binging.[19]
3. A purging reaction in order to counteract the effects of binging, which may include self-induced vomiting, laxative/diuretic abuse, periods of starvation, exercise, etc.
4. A feeling of loss of control around the binging/purging cycle.
5. Self-evaluation is unduly influenced by body shape and weight.
6. The disturbance does not occur exclusively during episodes of anorexia nervosa.

Compulsive (binge) eating/Binge Eating Disorder (BED)[20]

1. Preoccupation with food, and binge-eating episodes.
2. Lack of purging or other compensatory behavior.
3. Marked distress/guilt at the binge-eating episodes.

Eating disorders with clinical severity that do *not* fit either one of these three categories are included under the diagnosis Eating Disorder Not Otherwise Specified (EDNOS). The fact that EDNOS (the residual category) is necessary in clinical practice shows that there are types of eating disorders that cannot be easily differentiated. Atypical anorexia would include, for instance, a case where a female sufferer's menstrual cycle fails to stop, which may mean being denied the diagnosis of anorexia nervosa and, instead, end up

---

[18] DSM-IV notes that with bulimia "the binge eating and inappropriate compensatory behaviors both occur, on average, at least twice a week for 3 months." It further defines two subtypes of Bulimia Nervosa (1) the purging type, which involves self-induced vomiting or the misuse of laxatives, diuretics, or enemas, and (2) the non-purging type whereby the sufferer uses other inappropriate compensatory behaviors, including fasting or excessive exercise, but does not regularly engage in techniques used in purging-type bulimia.

[19] DSM-IV defines binging as: (1) eating, in a discrete period of time (e.g., within any two-hour period), an amount of food that is definitely larger than most people would eat during a similar period of time and under similar circumstances. If amounts or frequencies do not match the criteria then an Eating Disorder Not Otherwise Specified (EDNOS) may be diagnosed. And (2) a sense of lack of control over eating during the episode (e.g., a feeling that one cannot stop eating or control what or how much one is eating).

[20] The DSM-IV Criteria require binge eating behavior at least two days per week for six months, while the CDI does not specify the frequency.

categorized under EDNOS. This is recognized as a delicate problem, which the *New York Times* (November 13, 2004) addresses in the article "Sorry, Your Eating Disorder Doesn't Meet Our Criteria." This suggests that diagnoses do not only serve doctors in describing a problem, but may also be of substantial value for the patient.
Furthermore, the three eating disorders anorexia, bulimia and BED also sometimes merge: The majority of anorectics have binge-purging attacks, but bulimia can also develop into anorexia (Gerlinghoff and Backmund, 2004). In other words, diagnoses may be necessary for statistics and prognoses, but they force a blurry clinical picture to fit into distinct categories. This problem has been widely recognized and continues to be food for academic debate (Münsterman and Steins, 2003).

What does this mean for a study dealing with an online support group on eating disorders? It indicates that there is a discrepancy between people with severe eating or weight problems and the medical/diagnostic vocabulary to categorize them. The fact that this study focuses on the actual interaction of people outside of the medical sphere (namely a *peer* support group), means that it is highly problematic to assume that those people have a diagnosis. The dubious nature of eating disorder diagnoses could be referred to in an online support group, especially when a novice member introduces her/himself to the forum by means of her/his eating disorder diagnosis. The feminist cultural model offers an alternative to the medical model, which broadens the focus of diagnostic criteria and also sheds light on other aspects that play a role in eating disorders, such as the overwhelming majority of sufferers being women.

3.3 A solution: The cultural model of eating disorders

Since the early 1990s, feminist analysts such as Bordo (1995) and Orbach (2001) have been criticizing the established medical model for ignoring the role that culture plays in eating disorders. The medical model focuses on rigorously distinguishing between criteria and definitions of "anorectic-like behavior," "bulimic thinking," "weight-preoccupation" etc. (see previous section). Furthermore, it fails to offer a satisfying explanation for the fact that approximately 95% of those with eating disorders are female (e.g., Gerlinghoff and Backmund, 2004). Feminist scholars have argued that the medical model obscures the fact that culture has a *routine* grip on the female body, plus the model ignores the experiences of self-deprecation, self-hate, and shame that are so commonplace, especially among women (Bordo, 1995: 66). Therefore, Bordo proposed approaching eating disorders not from a pathological phenomenon angle, but from the perspective that they are located at the extreme of a social continuum in the pursuit of slenderness. Bordo thus has gone beyond the medical model and thereby explained that gender not only triggers or contributes to eating disorders (as in the medical model), but is "primary and productive" (Bordo, 1995: 54). For instance, the important symptom of a distorted body image (one of the criteria of the DSM-IV, see previous section) is not unique to anorectics, but typical for women in a westernized culture.[21]

The cultural model offers interpretations of the "slender body," where no primary distinction is made between the disordered body and any other body. Thus, it does not stick to the medical approach in which the body is seen as a "tabula rasa" upon which the disorder is inscribed, and which can only be deciphered by a medical expert. In the cultural model, getting an eating disorder does not just mean falling ill, but is seen as "an attempt to embody certain values, to create a body that will speak for the self in a meaningful and powerful way" (Bordo, 1995: 67). Eating disorders are then considered as a practice that is interpreted through a "set of interrelationships between knowledge, social practices and institutional authority" (Hepworth, 1999: 121). The cultural/feminist model can use this premise to explain that men *also* develop eating disorders. However, it primarily seeks to find the cultural values that can account for the fact that women are so much more susceptible to them. Bordo distinguished four of these values. The slender female body signifies:

1. The "promise of [the] transcendence of domestic femininity and admission to the privileged world, a world in which admiration is granted not to softness but to will, autonomy, and rigor" (Bordo, 1995: 68).
2. Taking up a smaller amount of space in the world.
3. Control over hunger, needs and desire (both practically and symbolically), which is internalized in shame over needs and appetites.
4. The ideal of "a perfectly managed and regulated self, within a consumer culture, which has made the actual management of hunger and desire intensely problematic" (Bordo, 1995: 68).

These values have also been labeled as the contradictory ideology of femininity, which is acted out (through eating, hungering, purging and exercise) upon the body: "The ideal of slenderness [...] and the diet and exercise regimens that have become inseparable from it, offer the illusion of meeting, through the body, the contradictory demands of the contradictory ideology of femininity" (Bordo, 1995: 172). Those with bulimia or BED, which are both characterized by binge episodes, often see the binging as the ultimate failure

[21] Bordo (1995: 56) relied on two studies which revealed that 75% to 95% of all women consider themselves too fat, or overestimate their body size.

of the embodiment of the two ideologies, because it expresses a loss of control. Purging or vomiting is the response to the shame and self-loathing that results from the binge.

In an attempt to link cultural ideology to the bodily self, Lester (1997) has proposed the concept of *self-technology* (Foucault, 1986), which offers a theorization of the embodied self (uniting the bodily and cultural self) as a fluid and dynamic entity that is shaped through the engagement in meaningful cultural practices. Thus, the anorectic's struggle can be read as an elaborate and sophisticated self-technology which has gone awry as a result of interrelated familial and cultural factors. Along a similar line, Gugutzer (2005) pointed out that eating disordered individuals have an identity problem, which includes extremely low self-esteem or even self-loathing, which they try to solve by means of their bodies. The eating, weight or beauty problems, i.e., the more observable aspects of eating disorders, are just symptoms. If the body is "controlled," sufferers feel better about, or sometimes even proud of themselves.

The cultural approach that goes beyond the medical conceptualization of eating disorders has frequently been confronted with the question of why only *some* women develop a full-blown eating disorder, despite the fact that *all* women are subject to the same cultural values. The answer is that people are not formed *solely* by their interactions with homogenizing images and ideologies concerning femininity. Rather, "[t]he unique configurations (of ethnicity, social class, sexual orientation, religion, genetics, education, family, age, and so forth) that make up each person's life will determine how each *actual* [person] is affected by our culture" (Bordo, 1995: 62, emphasis in original).

For the present study, the cultural model enables an understanding of eating disorders as a cultural phenomenon, and an online support group on eating disorders as one of the cultural settings in which eating disorders are negotiated, without being limited by medical definitions and criteria (hence, diagnoses). Moreover, it also implies and explains that many more women participate in these groups than men. Without wanting to focus on the participants' gender, the cultural model suggests that gender could be relevant in the accomplishment of eating disorders in an online forum.[22] In online settings, gender can be accomplished through nicknames (see also section 2.7).

---

[22] It must be made clear that from the proposed ethnomethodological point of view, the current study is not interested in a forum participant's "real" gender. Nevertheless, it may be presumed that the majority is female (cf. Leiberich et al., 2004).

3.4 Eating disorders as identity for diagnosed participants

In the previous sections, I have developed the view that we must distinguish between diagnoses of eating disorders (anorexia, bulimia, BED etc.) in the medical model and presenting oneself as eating disordered using a diagnosis in actual situations. I will consider some sociological theories of diagnosis in order to better understand the potential relevance of discussing eating disorders in terms of diagnoses in an online forum. Section 3.2 considered the basis upon which individuals commonly receive an eating disorder diagnosis. Two aspects about the social impact of diagnosis seem important for the present study. First, it has been noted that the number of subclinical cases of eating disorders is very high, which implies that many sufferers do not even get diagnosed. This phenomenon is looked at more closely in the next section. Second, socially speaking, diagnoses have both positive and negative consequences. In this section, I focus on the negative consequences of an eating disorder diagnosis (stigmatization) and the potential elevation of this burden in online support groups.

In the field of medical sociology, diagnoses have been discussed as a social construction (e.g., Blaxter, 1978; Brown, 1995). Blaxter (1978) distinguishes between diagnosis as a process, which includes the practitioner's imposing a diagnosis onto a patient, and diagnosis as a category, which refers to medical knowledge or nosology. In medical practice, diagnoses are crucial, since they have a prescriptive function for treatment (Blaxter, 1978). Moreover, a diagnosis has great value to the patient, since it provides personal, emotional control by way of learning the extent and nature of a particular ailment and it offers the legal basis for the provision of health services, welfare benefits, etc. (Brown, 1995). The positive side of diagnosis also has its contrary: Diagnosis can actually cause stigmatization (Goffman, 1986; Münsterman and Steins, 2003).

On a societal level, eating disorders are highly stigmatized. They are frequently portrayed in the media as the fashion diseases of girls who are striving to attain a top model beauty ideal via extreme dieting and *not* as serious psychiatric disorders (Schoemaker, 2002). It has been claimed that those with an eating disorder diagnosis find it difficult to manage their identities with stigmatization (Rich, 2006). For instance, significant others (family, peers, teachers, etc.) of anorectics appear to make sense of the eating disorder by focusing on *visual* aspects of weight loss and gain, and thus reduce it to a problem of pathology or irrationality. Stigmatization for those with bulimia is even worse than for anorectics. Münsterman and Steins (2003) revealed that someone who is considered a bulimic is ascribed stereotypes often associated with bulimia, which are seen far more negatively than the stereotypes associated with anorexia. While anorexia is often associated with perfectionism, discipline, control, seriousness, loneliness, rationality, etc., bulimia is characterized by traits such as loss of control, fear, failure to draw a boundary between the self and others, dependency, insecurity, depression, extreme mood swings, aggression and being chaotic. It can thus be said that the influence of stigmatization on those with eating orders in general is a serious problem. Furthermore, the stigmatization of those close to someone with an eating order is also strong, and can cause further problems in the patient's treatment with sometimes fatal results (Hohmeier, 1975). Hence, a diagnosis may be an acceptance of one's eating problems, but it can also cause stigmatization, which could lead to the patient ultimately denying the diagnosis.

The social stigma of eating disorders can be assumed to be diminished in an online support group. Recovery support groups and online forums are meant to be spaces that offer protection from social stigmatization because the members *share* a stigmatized problem (Johnson et al., 2002). Online communities are often considered to be even safer than "real life" self-help groups, since the absence of potentially discrediting visual cues prevents the "who is the thinnest" type of contest (Walstrom, 2000b). In other words, it is possible that the relation between diagnosis and stigma is minimized in online support groups, which implies that dealing with an eating disorder diagnosis is probably less difficult than in other social contexts.

Considerations of the social construction and stigma of the diagnosis inform an understanding of the "accomplishment of eating disorders" via the disclosing of one's diagnosis. However, it is essential to read the diagnoses as participants' constructions so that they are not merely taken at face value, because in numerous cases the actual problem does not fit into the official diagnostic criteria. Furthermore, it may be presumed that a diagnosis is usually less problematic in online contexts than in encounters with non-eating disordered individuals. However, the empirical study needs to illuminate the role of eating disorder diagnoses and norms involved in an online support group.

3.5 Eating disorders as identity for undiagnosed participants

It can be assumed that the number of subclinical cases of eating disorders is extremely high (Gerlinghoff and Backmund, 2004; Van Hoeken et al., 2005). Unreported cases of bulimia are estimated to consist of as much as *two-thirds* of the total number clinical cases (Karwauts, 1997). A German study of subclinical cases involving 740 students between the ages of 12 and 32 revealed that early signals of eating disorders could be determined for many of the study's participants (Aschenbrenner, 2001). Approximately 29% of the women and 13% of the men in the study reported chronic dieting, fasting days, purging, binging, excessive exercise or use of appetite suppressants, laxatives or dehydrators. This confirmation of the gap between "true" cases and medically diagnosed cases is the first indication that having an eating disorder is not as simple as having an eating disorder diagnosis. Instead, many people with eating problems do not (or only much later) decide to seek medical help, or drop out of the medical treatment program before they have fully recovered. While the potential relevance of diagnosis for eating disorders in an online support group was noted in the previous section, this section explores the potential relevance of *not* having an eating disorder diagnosis. This is important, because these online groups are also designed to reach individuals who have not yet managed to find medical assistance, and thus are still undiagnosed. The barriers to seeking medical help are possibly smaller for *online* support groups involving eating disorders. There are at least three interrelated explanations for the thresholds involved in medical consultations: The social stigma, the gradual development of eating disorders and the problem of compliance.

A. Social stigma of symptoms

In section 3.4, I looked at how an eating disorder *diagnosis* could be experienced as a potential stigma. However, symptoms of disordered eating (before medical help is sought and the patient is diagnosed) can also be described as a stigma, more precisely as a *discreditable* (hidden) stigma (see 2.4). In fact, the early phases of these disorders are often characterized by the hiding of one's symptoms for various reasons, but possibly in part due to stigma or the feeling that one is being irrational. Sufferers may pretend they have eaten much more than they really have, wear oversized clothes in order to hide their thin bodies, etc. Meanwhile, the role of stigma in cases of bulimia is considered to be serious, since the loss of control a bulimic encounters while binging and vomiting or purging can cause immense feelings of shame (Gugutzer, 2005). After the diagnosis of bulimia was implemented in 1980, the number of cases of bulimia increased erratically (Habermas, 2000), which suggests that the fear of disclosure of these shameful symptoms to a medical practitioner was even stronger in the past. A retrospective interview study confirmed that bulimia sufferers began feeling that they could actually seek help in the medical system in 1980 (Habermas, 1992). However, the stigma of specific eating disorder symptoms may still be a reason why sufferers would be reluctant to approach professionals. It is possible that the level of shame and stigma is significantly reduced in online support groups.

B. The gradual development of eating disorders

Eating disorders usually start with a diet and gradually develop into an eating disorder. Thirty-five percent of "normal dieters" become pathological dieters, and of that 35%, 20-25% eventually acquire partial or full-syndrome eating disorders (Shisslak et al., 1995). This implies that dieters need to recognize the seriousness of their problems before they (or their caretakers, teachers, etc.) decide for them that medical help is necessary. The gradual onset of the symptoms may complicate the identification of a particular eating disorder. As long as sufferers fail to visit a health provider, they fall under the statistical category of subclinical cases, even if the disordered eating has long ago turned into an eating disorder. It could be that these individuals join an online support group to figure out whether they have an eating disorder or not.

C. Motivation problem linked to "eating disorder identity"

Another reason for not seeking professional help may be related to personal motivation. A very frequent problem in clinical practice regarding patients with eating disorders is the issue of compliance or motivation, also called "readiness to change" (Treasure et al., 2005: 104). The patient may not be able to distance her/himself from the anorectic identity, or the eating disorder identity (e.g., Bruch, 2001; Lock et al., 2004; Malson, 1998). This identification with the eating disorder has also been called the parasite of anorexia that has replaced the self (Epston, 2000).[23] The following quotation from an interview with an anorectic woman illustrates this point:

> But I am the anorexia. This is my identity [...] it has actually become my identity, and I think that's that's the problem with it. I think it becomes (.) can become an all-consuming identity (Malson, 1998: 147).

In this light, recovering from an eating disorder has been described as a process of coming to sense the "real" self (Reindl, 2001). Accordingly, re-initiating the process of developing the self is one of the general aims of psychotherapy regarding anorectic women (Orbach, 2001). This implies that recovery demands a sufferer has to learn to "put into words" the experiences that were once "put into body." But since "words are as, if not more, problematic for women with eating disorders than their relationship to food" (Farrell, 1995: xiv), the readiness, or motivation to leave one's eating disorder identity behind requires that the sufferer have a sense of resolute decisiveness and endurance. Concretely, s/he may not be willing or ready to "give up" restricted eating and accept a weight gain, which are requirements to the receiving of treatment in the first place, since the psyche is too disturbed to engage in therapy when the body is in a state of severe emaciation (Bruch, 2001). Thus, one reason that sufferers may end up refraining from seeking

[23] In medical terms, this phenomenon is called *egosyntonicity*. It refers to the sense that the anorexia nervosa is part of the self (Treasure et al., 2005), which is felt by many sufferers.

medical assistance or refusing treatment may have to do with the fact that they nevertheless experience the eating disorder as a positive identity and are not ready yet to sever their relation to it (Tan et al., 2003).

To conclude, we can expect members of online support groups who are too ashamed to seek medical help, others who do not fully comprehend the severity of their eating problems and those who refuse medical treatment altogether. At the same time, it is possible that some participants are just "ordinary" dieters and are not "really" eating disordered at all. These aspects may be significant for those entering an online forum on eating disorders. However, the resistance towards therapy or the medical system as a whole has another important appearance in the field of eating disorders: *Pro-ana* (pro-anorexia) and *pro-mia* (pro-bulimia).

3.6 *Pro*-eating disorders as identity in online support groups

Motivation or compliance is a medical concept, not a patient's perspective. Conrad (1985) has offered "another look at compliance" through the observation that patients may have very good reasons to resist treatment. For instance, medication may require a reorganization of life, which the individual may not be willing to conduct. The condition may thus end up being preferred to treatment. This is an argument to use the term *self-regulation* rather than compliance (Conrad, 1985). For eating disorders, the possibility that individuals prefer self-regulating their problem is found in the pro-eating disorders (pro-ana and pro-mia) movement.

Sufferers of eating disorders who are not ready or willing to undergo treatment may turn to virtual places that are free from the usual social stigmatization and pressure to undergo treatment, which consists of a considerable number of pro-ana and pro-mia websites. I will now focus on pro-ana, since there has been very little research conducted on pro-mia to date. At first sight, the primary purpose of pro-ana sites seems to be the celebration and promotion of anorexia as a lifestyle. They frequently show the emaciated bodies of anorectics and offer fashion accessories to foster a sense of community. In related chat-rooms and forums, users can exchange information and their ideas on anorexia-related topics. They provide and receive motivation and "how to" advice, including ideas on low-calorie intake and avoidance, distractions from hunger, etc. Although the real prevalence of pro-ana sites is impossible to determine, it has been estimated that it exceeds 500 in the US alone (Chesley et al., 2003), but today this number is probably much higher (ca. 400 in the Netherlands according to *De Volkskrant* 03.05.08). The dominant opinion about pro-ana and its related online communities is that they present dangerous information and are thus a risk, especially to adolescents and young adults (Norris et al., 2006). There has been heated debate in line with this about the closing down of these sites in the US. This has been rejected as a solution by the Academy for Eating Disorders, however, arguing that, despite the troublesome content, it is better to resist the pro-movement by using other means (Schoemaker, 2002). However, France made it a crime in April 2008 to distribute pro-ana information.

Nevertheless, in some critical publications, the pro-ana sites are read as spaces "where women who are struggling with anorexia can potentially find sanctuary from the surveillance and regulatory mechanisms of control in the public sphere" (Dias, 2003: 1). Dias has criticized clinical practice for dividing sufferers into the compliant and resistant categories (or, "good" and "bad"), which she interpreted as a reinforcement of hegemonic binaries used to historically pathologize and silence women. Drawing on poststructuralist feminist accounts of subversion and contradiction in anorexia (Bordo, 1995; Grosz, 1994), she categorized pro-ana as a type of resistance. Fox et al. (2005) have also emphasized that the pro-ana movement does not use the Internet solely as a medium for communication and information sharing, but also as a platform to reject and resist mainstream models of health and illness. Pro-ana should not be seen as a lifestyle, then, but as a form of self-regulation, or a coping mechanism, which is a response to social and emotional difficulties. The pro-anorexia movement similarly does not merely promote anorexia, but advocates and gives advice on damage limitation and survival strategies to *reduce* the risks associated with extremely low weight.

Although in various media and medical discourses, pro-ana is depicted as irrational and distorted and as promoting a deadly disease, Dias (2003) has pointed to the fact that the voices of these women themselves are rarely heard. She discovered that users of these sites may display their ambivalence towards both the pro-ana and the medical views, which suggests that the main differences between the two camps are more of an enforced interpretation by outsiders. This suggestion is confirmed by various other sources. For instance, a recovery forum on eating disorders was closed due to what was described as its destructive nature (Johnson et al., 2002). The formal description of "recovery forum" apparently does not guarantee that the forum is beneficial to actual recovery. Consider also the following excerpt, which comes from an interview between a researcher and a pro-ana website owner.

> Q: Many of your sites have links to pro-recovery websites... Do you find that even pro-recovery websites can be triggering, or helpful in maintaining your disorder?

> A: Yes… as a matter of fact, the first site i went to was [XX]. By far that is the most triggering site I've been to, its made by an EX-anorexic. And it's a RECOVERY site. I learned more from that site than any PRO site could offer
>
> Source: Dias (2003: 16).

On the other hand, most pro-anorectics do not tend to see recovery negatively; instead, they feel that they are not ready to lay down the "eating disorder security blanket" (Dias, 2003: 20) just yet. They live with a conflict between needing the eating disorder and wanting to survive, and until they have gained a "readiness to change" (see 3.5) they remain pro-ana. This "defense" of pro-ana sites and forums clearly does not argue with the purpose of proliferating eating disorders, but with the intention not to deny anorectics spaces where they can "meet, free from judgment, to support each other and break the isolation" (Dias, 2003: 20).

Some studies do not recognize that the pro-ana and contra-ana (= pro-recovery) positions are quite diffuse and blurred, as I just argued. Lyons et al. (2006) distinguished the two groups per definition and concluded that pro-anorectics and recovering anorectics basically differ in the language they use in their online forums and message boards. The language used by the pro-anorectics indicated, among other things, a reduced level of cognitive processing and a lower degree of self-preoccupation. The researchers of this study have suggested that the pro-anorectics' language use hints at a coping strategy aimed at stabilizing them emotionally (i.e., by giving them a sense of control over their own illness), which could explain their resistance to psychological treatment. One problem with this kind of research is that language use is treated as a one-to-one display or representation of cognitive processes and states, rather than as the conduct of actions in a specific setting. But the main problem is that the identity of the participants is defined a priori and not approached as an accomplishment. Since a dichotomy between the pros and contras is presumed, it is only the contradictions between the two groups that can be articulated, not those between members or within single members' contributions. Therefore, in the present study, it is not presumed that only "contra-eating disorder" identities are articulated in online support groups or recovery forums; rather, the analysis is sensitive to both pro and contra identities, although pro-identities are probably rare in forums that are positioned as supportive of medical treatment.

3.7 Community and identity matter: Previous research on online eating disorder support groups

Previous studies of online forums or support groups on eating disorders have not focused on identity or community aspects and have instead tended to concentrate on the discursive practices linked to support (Johnson et al., 2002; Winzelberg, 1997), how the forum interaction is experienced (Leiberich et al., 2004), how communication may create safety and thus serve the therapeutic potential (Walstrom, 2000b). I will review these studies in more detail to map out the state of the art of research of online support groups on eating disorders.

Most of the studies discussed the positive relation between online forum participation and medical treatment. Leiberich et al. (2004) found that the analyzed online forum (*Hungrig-Online*, the forum also analyzed here) functions as a favorable supplement to therapy. Moreover, online communities may improve compliance to therapy regimens (Celio et al., 2002). According to Winzelberg (1997), participating in forums may serve in lieu of professional treatment, whereas Leiberich et al. (2004) found that patients with eating disorders are encouraged to undergo therapy as a result of the support and understanding they receive from their Internet peers. The role of professionals in those forums is not always discussed. However, Johnsen et al. (2002) found the interactions in a forum on eating disorders to be destructive (in contrast to online forums dealing with other kinds of disorders), which caused them to recommend greater professional involvement in these forums.

Leiberich et al. (2004) evaluated the largest German website on eating disorders by means of a questionnaire. It was discovered that 79.7% of the respondents expected to receive information regarding other self-help options, access to appropriate therapy or information on other types of therapy. Furthermore, 24.4% hoped for a rapid recovery process as a result of information received, while 47.5% sought comfort from their peers and 48.1% reported having found satisfactory support via the electronic exchange. In the area of the exchange of experiences, 35.9% reported feeling reassured to know that other people had the same problems. The researchers did not refrain from pointing out that their research did not measure the levels of actual use of these websites and companion forums. This is important to note since what people assert they do on a questionnaire and what they actually do can vary widely (i.e., a well-known validity problem).

Information on what participants of an online support group on eating disorders actually *do* in the messages they post, is offered by Winzelberg's (1997) discourse analysis of 306 messages from a US forum on eating disorders, collected over a period of three months. He found that 31% of the messages involved self-disclosure, followed by requests for information (23%) and the direct provision of emotional support (16%).[24] The results indicate that participants of this support group used the same assistance strategies as face-to-face group members. Winzelberg admitted, however, that there were many messages that included content that was appropriate to more than one category.[25] Furthermore, he did not examine the exchange of postings between members. The only point he made related to interaction is that inaccurate and potentially dangerous information (12% of all information provided) was in many cases corrected by other group members. It remains unclear why Winzelberg coded information "inaccurate and outside the standards of medical and psychological care," just as it remains unclear how participants responded to the corrections of inaccurate information.

Walstrom (2000b) conducted a qualitative discourse analysis of interactions in a US forum on eating disorders. She discovered that the information and support that are offered exceed the inquiries by the initiator of a thread, but also that the interaction "orients to" (at least) two norms. The first norm involves the systematic, extensive use of facework (see 2.3) and the second entails standards for displaying physical appearances, which implies the disclosure of only very general information about body sizes. Although these norms may be assumed to be "community norms," Walstrom did not go into the issue of community as such. However, in the analysis of her data, she has implicitly addressed it. Consider the following excerpt, an initial posting composed by novice member Karla.

> I've been to this [*sic*] a few times – I always seems [*sic*] to feel extra self-concious [*sic*] in groups, because I feel like everyone is judging the extent of my sickness on my appearance. If I feel fat one day, I feel guilty for claiming to have an eating disorder. If I restrict for a while, then I feel more sick and more eligible for the title of 'eating disordered' […]
>
> Source: Walstrom (2000b: 767-768).

This excerpt demonstrates Karla considers the label (*'eating disordered'*) neither a diagnosis nor a generally stigmatized label, but something one has to be eligible for. In other words, the title of eating disordered is an accountable identity that requires legitimacy. Karla contends that being in a group makes this accountability even more intense, which implies that even in an online

[24] Other content categories were Support Requested, Information Provided, Disclosure Requested and the category "Other," which included friendship and board maintenance (Winzelberg, 1997).

[25] This "coding" problem is inevitable in quantitative studies and is addressed in section 1.3.

community, the *title of 'eating disordered'* must be legitimized. Walstrom stated:

> This [excerpt] reveals that support group participation status is an accomplishment rather than an inherent right. Karla's use of the honorary term 'title' and quotation marks around 'eating disordered' stresses the positive nature and value that she attributes to claiming an eating disorder identity, ostensibly as a basis for support group participant status (2000b: 768).

Thus, Walstrom's data and analysis give a first indication of the role of membership and community status regarding the interactions that take place in an online eating disorder support group. Apparently, it is relevant that the label "eating disordered" or an eating disorder diagnosis is considered an identity, but the question also rises whether the concern with accountability is related to the fact that Karla is a novice member who is posting for the first time. These are the issues the empirical analysis will focus on (see part 2).

3.8 Conclusion

In this chapter it has been argued that a study of the discourse of entering an online community on eating disorders must be attentive to various identity aspects, which are socially relevant to eating disorders. It can be expected that, in the case of online support groups on eating disorders, some members have gotten a diagnosis, or are engaged in therapy, whereas others are undiagnosed. For this reason, I propose approaching eating disorders from a cultural model, rather than a medical one because of its arguable basis in diagnoses.

Eating disorder diagnoses have been discussed for their potential importance in online communities. The problem of eating disorder diagnoses is that they are (possibly inevitably) imprecise or ambiguous. A diagnosis brings relief to the patient in the sense that s/he knows what is wrong, and further legitimizes her/him for medical care, but at the same time, it has been found that eating disorder diagnoses are highly stigmatized, particularly bulimia.

The apparently huge number of undiagnosed or subclinical sufferers of eating disorders could imply that it is especially these types of individuals who engage in online communities, as they have no therapeutic space in which to discuss their problems. Various explanations for eating disordered people who do not seek medical help have been discussed. The social stigma may be a barrier for seeking help to some, but the gradual development of an eating disorder and a lack of "readiness to change" also seem to play a role. It may be that these factors, which stand in the way of medical consultation, are less of a threshold for seeking support in an online forum. If this is true, the question is whether they still play a role in the online support group.

Individuals with eating disorders who refuse treatment can engage in the pro-ana, pro-mia or otherwise pro-eating disorders movement. A review of literature on this movement resulted in an unstable and unclear distinction between pro- and contra-eating disorder engagements or identities. Therefore, the present study is sensitive to both pro- and contra-identities in online support groups and conceptually approaches both as accomplishments.

Finally, I reviewed previous studies of online support groups on eating disorders. In most of these studies, these groups are considered basically beneficial (either as a supplement to or replacement for medical treatment, or as increasing motivation to seek treatment). Walstrom (2000b) provides the present study with an incentive, since the interaction in a US forum suggests that community indeed plays a role in establishing one's participation in such a forum. A novice member in this forum "orients to" the title of "eating disordered" (which could also be a diagnosis) as something one must earn, not in general, but particularly in groups, hence, also in online communities. Thus, the reviewed literature on eating disorders offers some reason to expect that in the process of entering an online support group on eating disorders, community and connected identities become particularly significant in the context of this particular, stigmatized problem.

Part II
Discourse analysis

Chapter 4

Research design: The forum, ethics, data and method

4.1 Introduction

The aim of the analysis is to examine the situation when new participants enter an online forum on eating disorders, especially with regard to the extent to which participants "orient to" identities and being a community. In this chapter, I present my chosen methodological approach. This is an analysis of interaction, which is grounded in ethnomethodological stances, discourse analysis and conversation analysis. Moreover, I describe the data selection, which delivered the material for the microanalysis of 27 forum threads (see 4.4 and 5.5).

As I have argued, community, or the accomplishment of community in an online forum, is framed by structural features of a Community of Practice, such as system design, association structure and forum rules. These issues need to be explored as context knowledge for the analysis of the ways members discursively enter a community.[26] Therefore, I describe these general features of the analyzed forum in section 4.2. Subsequently, the ethical questions that inevitably rise in this type of research on a sensitive community like a forum on eating disorders are considered in section 4.3.

4.2 The *Hungrig-Online* forum

The selected forum is available through the website of the German association *Hungrig-Online* (HO) (Hungry-Online). I will describe the forum and the HO association on the basis of texts and documents from the HO website (including Rules and Regulations, self-descriptions of HO available through the site, press releases, etc.). Moreover, I also draw on survey studies on the use and users of the forum (Kral and Presslich, 2002; Leiberich et al., 2004), the outcomes of which have also been summarized *in* the HO forum itself (Leiberich, 2005, December 23), also referred to as "survey 2003." This exploratory description can be seen as part of the *frame* of the forum conversa-

[26] In other words, a discourse analysis requires an ethnographic investigation of the HO setting to recognize the importance of certain activities, but also the use of certain terms (Koole, 1997).

tions (see 1.5 and 1.6). Hence, this section sets out to describe the characteristics of a Community of Practice that must be considered as background information to the interaction analysis. *Hungrig-Online*, which offers both information and communication possibilities, is grounded in the following motivation:

> Anorexie, Bulimie, beiden ist eines gemeinsam: sie bleiben lange Zeit verborgen, die/der Betroffene möchte es mit sich selbst ausmachen. Wir bieten eine Alternative zum einsamen Schweigen! Das Internet ist oft die erste Informationsquelle und auch die erste Anlaufstelle. Auf diesen Seiten sollen von Magersucht oder Fress-/Brechsucht Betroffene und deren Angehörige die Möglichkeit haben, sich zu informieren und mit anderen ins Gespräch zu kommen. (http://www.hungrig-online.de/content/view/ 27/27/)
>
> [Anorexia, bulimia, both have one [thing] in common: They remain secrets for a long time, which means that the sufferer often wishes to deal with it alone. We offer an alternative to the lonely silence! The Internet is frequently the first source of information and also the first contact point. Those who struggle with anorexia and bulimia, and their relatives are offered the opportunity on these websites to find information and get in touch with others.]

The objective of offering a contact point or place of refuge, as an alternative to being isolated with eating problems is thus central to HO's profile. This renders it particularly important to understand how the sufferers' silence is broken and interaction is initiated. This motivation has been reformulated repeatedly since the founding of HO. At the time the collected threads were produced, people with the disorders of Binge Eating Disorders and Obesity were also added as part of the target audience, but also the following sentences were added:

> Das Angebot von Hungrig-Online.de kann und soll keine Therapie ersetzen. Unser Ziel ist es vielmehr, durch Aufklärung und Information ein Bewußtsein für diese Essstörungen zu schaffen und Unterstützung und Motivation bei der Suche nach Hilfe zu bieten. (http://www.hungrig-online.de/)
>
> [The services of Hungrig-Online cannot and should not be a substitute for treatment. Rather, it is our objective to establish awareness of eating disorders through education and information and to offer support and motivation for those seeking help.]

Hence, HO makes it clear that it does not offer therapy, and views its task as one of motivating its members to seek professional help.

The development of the HO forum

In 1999, the website *Hungrig-Online* was launched by a physician, Dr. Jan Nedoschill at the Department Children and Youth Psychiatry in the Academic Hospital Erlangen. He and Wolfgang Gawlik, the founder of a similar website (www.magersucht-online.de), whose partner suffered from an eating disorder, decided to cooperate and combine their two websites. The original purpose of the new site was to provide information on the various kinds of eating disorders, but in 2000, the forum was added to the website as a space for sufferers to offer and receive support.

In the beginning, the forum was comprised of seven sub-forums to specific topics, which were further differentiated over subsequent years, resulting in 17 peer sub-forums on topics of interest such as *Neu Hier* ("new here"), *Essverhalten* ("eating behavior"), *Ursachen* ("causes"), *Partnerschaft* ("relationships"), *Therapie* ("therapy"), *Buchempfehlungen* ("book recommendations"), etc. For an impression of its interface, see figure 1. Furthermore, the forum offers a range of sub-forums for professional advice (on therapies, clinics, medication, etc.), and the forum archive.[27] The forum is only one component of the total HO website's services which also includes online self-help groups, chat sessions, mailinglists, as well as extensive information which makes the site a well equipped and expansive area in the German field of eating disorders. In the forum, all postings have been archived since 2000. The archive is, just as the forum, publicly available to readers/lurkers without registration. Since 2000, over 939,000 contributions have been posted by over 23,000 participants to the forum alone.

[27] This description is based on HO's state of the art in February 2008.

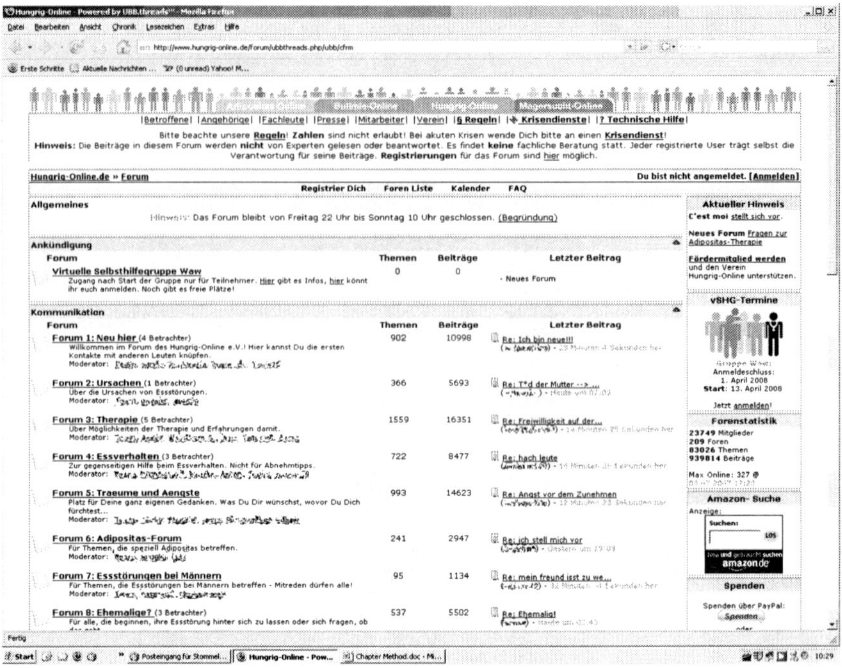

Fig. 1. Screen view of the HO forum (nicknames are made illegible)

HO's staff is comprised of those who are medically involved with eating disorders, and (ex-) sufferers or those who are otherwise familiar with eating disorders. All staff members are volunteers at HO. The association is build up around the following functions: Team head, medical-psychological head, technical head, staff manager, forums coordinator, head of the mailinglist for relatives, head of the mailinglist for sufferers, head of the chat, chief editor and chief service department. Those who occupy these positions also participate in forum conversations, which is obvious to other participants because her/his nickname is accompanied by her/his HO position. In other words, working for HO implies carrying an official label in the forum, which is perceivable in forum participation.

Objectives of the HO forum

A short portrait that has been available on the HO website since 2001, presents the objectives of the HO association.[28] HO wants to make sure that:

[28] See: http://web.archive.org/web/20050213142302/www.hungrig-online.de/presse/presseinformationen/kurzportrait.htm.

- Eating disordered individuals have access to a service, which will enable them to leave behind their social isolation. They need to be motivated to obtain information about their disorders and treatment options. The exchange with other sufferers or ex-sufferers is an additional form of support.
- Sufferers are encouraged to seek professional help, and the HO clinic database may be of use in this regard.
- Society, mainly the relatives and friends of eating disordered people, but also interested lay people are "enlightened" about eating disorders and HO thus offers public awareness about these disorders.

The value of the forum is first in its insistence on anonymity.[29] The anonymity is seen as especially important for sufferers who have not yet disclosed their problem, and therefore, have not yet taken steps to deal with the disorder. For them, anonymity secures the first and most important step to actually seek help. In general, HO seems to want to reach those people who have an eating disorder, but have not yet sought out or found professional treatment. They see eating disorders as particularly isolating, and therefore, see sufferers as critically cut off from help options. This renders the online basis of HO not only a simple alternative to an *offline* information centre, treatment centre or self-help group, but it also offers a surplus value. Because it is anonymously consultable and easily reachable for any German-speaking person with Internet access, it has a low-threshold character.

The question of whether HO is beneficial in the eating disorder recovery process is hard to answer. One of the outcomes of the survey held in 2003 (see below) is that, although the majority of the respondents claimed it had a positive effect, for more than one-third of the respondents nothing substantial changed since joining the forum, and approximately 25% said that their personal situation had remained very difficult; 18.2% experienced severe relapses of the eating disorder, while 12% complained of the development or aggravation of other psychic disorders. The 2003 survey, however, also showed that since initiating participation in HO, more positive than negative developments were reported among the participants concerning the eating disorder and psychic health (although evidently a causal relation cannot be determined). Positive developments include, for example, greater inner stability, increased acceptance of the eating disorder, increased ability to deal with the eating disorder and finding new acquaintances and friends.

---

[29] HO press information from 15.09.2002 at: http://web.archive.org/web/20040930202946/www.hungrig-online.de/presse/pressemitteilungen/HO_Sept_OnlineStudie.pdf.

The participants

It is difficult to determine the actual number of HO members. In January 2007, there were 21,386 registered members, but this number is misleading, since 13,789 of the registered users have never posted a contribution, which leaves more than 7000 active members. This number must be further nuanced, since, within a random 40-hour period (early January 2007) "only" 181 members produced a posting, within one week 300 members, within one month 574 members and in the course of one year (roughly 2006) 1526 members. Who are these active members? The 2003 survey received filled-out questionnaires from approximately 1,000 participants, of which 97% were female, 15% were under 18 years of age, 30% between 18 and 22, 32% between 22 and 30, and 13% over 30.

The major types of eating disorders (based on self-assessment) noted were anorexia and bulimia (anorexia 39%, bulimia 34.5% and "anorectic bulimia" 20.3%).[30] It is remarkable that approximately 40% of the respondents had never been diagnosed with an eating disorder before. The researchers concluded that this means that for many users, HO is the first step towards seeking help (information and communication) *before* they consult a medical practitioner. This conclusion was already drawn from a survey conducted in 2001 (Kral and Presslich, 2002). On the other hand, the 2003 survey concludes that HO is mainly used by long-term eating disordered individuals who consider the HO forum to be a sort of "Cape-of-Good-Hope," since earlier efforts and initiatives to find a cure had thus far failed, or had not yielded desired results. The actual state of the participants' eating disorders is captured in symptom frequencies the week before the questionnaire was filled out. Episodes of binge eating were the most common (54.4 %), vomiting was almost as common (49.8%) and food refusal as well (44.4%). Remarkably, 21.7% inflicted self-injury, known for its co-morbidity with eating disorders.[31]

After registering on the forum, 28.2% of the respondents started a form of treatment (ambulant or stationary therapy). Only 7.9% assumed they did not need any therapy after joining the HO forum. The HO association has declared that it is pleased with the results, since the objective of the forum is not to replace therapy, but to motivate and encourage members to seek therapy.

---

[30] HO staff, in fact, assumes that the majority of HO members are bulimic and not anorectic (personal communication with Wolfgang Gawlik). This can possibly be explained by the fact that bulimia is more stigmatized than anorexia (see section 3.4), and thus something that is more likely to be denied or hidden.

[31] Other research indicates that repeated self-harm through cutting, burning and overdosing occurs in approximately 15-25% of clinic samples (Favaro and Santonastaso, 1997).

What are the participants' major objectives? Based on the 2003 survey, Leiberich et al. (2004) pointed out that most participants sought information about their symptoms and support in their assessment of themselves as either "ill" or "unproblematic." Furthermore, the participants hoped that they would be better able to explain the cause and the background of their eating disorder when they talked about it with others. Others hoped that they would find self-help options, information about admission to treatment centers and the types of treatment, as well as a rapid cure and consolation. In 2001, it seems that of all participants who had ever initiated a topic, 70% perceived responses from other participants as constructive (Kral and Presslich, 2002). In 2003, almost 50% claimed to feel supported by the forum exchange through HO.

Finally, it is important to stress that anyone can use the HO forum; it is not limited solely to sufferers. The forum contains a special sub-forum for relatives and other concerned individuals, but these members are equally free to contribute to any forum thread.

Design of the forum

Reading forum threads is possible without registration, but for active participation one needs to register. There is the option to choose a nickname, but when this is not chosen, the login name will appear in postings. Moreover, participants can choose to add a profile, a place of residence, a profession, hobbies, date of birth and various other online addresses (Skype, ICQ). Notably, the type of eating disorder and sex/gender are not included on the profile form. Furthermore, the forum does not offer the option of creating an avatar, which is a picture linked to the nickname of the participant.

In the forum design, no strict differentiation is made between sufferers from the various disorders, which implies that anorectics can receive advice from bulimics and support from obese participants. However, there are a few sub-forums (of the 17) that focus on special groups: An obesity forum, an "otherwise concerned" forum (*Angehoerige*), an ex-sufferers forum and an eating disorders and men's forum.

In order to take part in forum discussions, one either responds to current threads or begins a new thread. The creator of a thread gives the thread a title, which appears on the forum's first interface. Readers decide whether they are interested in reading a particular thread based on its title.

The forum distinguishes between the statuses of members. For the first 30 posted contributions, the participant is considered a "new member." The effect may be that other participants will realize they are dealing with a novice member and will therefore be a little kinder, more tolerant or more likely to explain things than with experienced members. After 30 postings, a user is simply labeled "member." There are no further distinctions after this point among active members. The value of these status levels is minimal for the forum archive. The reason for this is that when something in the member's status changes, the change will be retroactively accomplished for all contributions ever posted by this participant. Hence, the fact that a participant was a "new member" or a "member" *at the time of posting* cannot be retraced after the participant has become "unregistered." Moreover, if a member became a moderator in 2004 and she maintains her original nickname, her postings thereafter would all be labeled "moderator." As a result, the only members with a status in archive postings that can be considered reliable is the status of "new member" of whom it is certain that s/he has not posted more than 30 times to the forum, and that s/he was still a novice at the time of posting.

The Rules and Regulations

In general, HO prescribes a polite and factual atmosphere of communication in the forum, and although serious critique on a factual level is encouraged, insulting, dishonorable, or aggressive behavior towards others is not allowed. Users are expected to be fair and engaged, and to be careful of their choice of words.

I will briefly consider the most important Rules and Regulations for participants who wish to contribute to the forum.[32] The most important rules are related to information in postings, which may harm or encourage other participants to increase their eating disordered behavior. This includes information about amounts of food, but also detailed descriptions of eating and purging behavior, weight quotations, BMI, but also, for example, a bra's cup size or one's grades in school. The reason is that numbers may lead to competition. Low weight may encourage emulation, panics, or further food denial; low calorie counts may lead to a phobia regarding food. It is for this same reason that it is forbidden to circumscribe weight (for example "limit of being critically underweight" or "extremely overweight"). Only the indications "underweight," "overweight" and "normal weight" are permitted.

There are more rules concerning the content of postings. For instance, suicidal thoughts, descriptions of self-injury, excessive narrations regarding sexuality and postings dealing with medical details and symptoms are not permitted. With regard to nicknames, it is stated that participation under more than one pseudonym is not desired since one could then create various different "identities," which would confuse other users. The HO association has also set some limits to the nicknames themselves. The forum rules state that a pseudonym may not be of an offensive, confusing, insinuating, or acrimonious nature or be identical to that of another participant, institution,

---

[32] See the current rules at: http://www.hungrig-online.de/content/view/34/31/. The rules as formulated in the beginning of 2005 were slightly different and can be found at: http://web.archive.org/web/20050209014621/www.hungrig-online.de/fregeln.htm.

or registered brand. What is understood as offensive, confusing, insinuating, or acrimonious is left implicit. It is not uncommon for a nickname to be rejected on the basis of this rule. The novice member is then directed to choose another nickname.

It appears that new participants are frequently not aware of the rules, which makes the intervention of moderators in the "New Here" sub-forum a common practice.[33] A moderator may, for example, replace the amounts of food quoted with asterisks: "I ate ** and felt really bad." In general, I have not come across any cases of an intentional violation of this rule. It appeared that when detailed information was posted unintentionally even other participants in their response advised the (novice) member to obscure or delete the sensitive information.[34] The 2003 survey revealed that a large majority of respondents accept the rules because a community simply needs rules to function, or because they value them as security. By contrast, less than 10% thought the rules were restrictive and limited their individual self-expression.

The forum moderators

Although it is indicated in the Users Information file that not all postings are read before they are placed, it appears that most postings are moderated when rules are violated. This job is carried out by the forum moderators, who are primarily ex-sufferers. Moderators also participate in the forum discussions, sometimes as participants with similar problems, sometimes more as advisers. In serious cases, the HO's medical staff may even reply to certain postings. Moderation is very important for the forum, since the experience is that unregulated conversations can cause harm. As a result, the moderators, in principle, need to be online 24 hours a day. Since this became too difficult during weekends, HO decided to close the forum on weekends. The sincerity of the HO association is thereby very well illustrated.

The 2003 survey revealed that more than 70% of the respondents support the moderators' right to guard the forum's communication rules, whereas only 9.8% disagreed. Furthermore, it appeared that the work of the moderators is appreciated:

---

[33] See for instance: http://www.hungrig-online.de/cgi-bin/ultimatebb.cgi?ubb=get_topic;f=165;t=000500

[34] Correcting your own postings seems to be a relatively frequent practice in the forum; hence, words can literally be taken back.

- Moderators give good advice: 53.6%.
- Moderators are experienced and very important attendants/tutors: 42.9%.
- Moderators are mostly too strict and focused on the rules: 9.7%.
- Moderators often think they know better: 12.9%.
- Moderators are very empathetic and comprehend the users' problems fairly well: 34.1%.
- Moderators are unnecessary and unhelpful: 0.0%.
- Moderators frequently write postings dealing with the fact that they personally struggle with a sickness or eating disorder: 9.1%.

The elaborate introduction of the HO forum seems necessary to form a basis for an understanding of the various aspects that may be relevant to novice members who enter the online group.

4.3 Ethical considerations and consequences

The sensitivity of the topic and vulnerability of sufferers of eating disorders requires a critical consideration of the ethics for an analysis of the interaction in the forum. In fact, in planning to engage in the research of online material, a consideration of the ethics is inevitably the first item to look at. Controversies and dilemmas on how to ethically conduct online research are part of today's practice (e.g., Buchanan, 2004). Many scholars, including Lawson, underline that "ethical Internet research is not merely a matter of following a series of guidelines, but of individual researchers' ongoing commitment to protect CMC participants/research subjects from harm" (2004: 95). The Association of Internet Research (AoIR) is probably the most authoritative voice that has formulated ethical recommendations for conducting Internet research (Ess and AoIR, 2002). In this section, I consider how these and other researchers deal with the issue of ethics for the purpose of establishing an ethically sound approach for the study at hand. The research material consists of nicknames and thread interactions. On the basis of Internet research ethics, I argue that, in the case of this research project, nicknames and interactions need to be studied in separate data collections. For both however, it must be stressed that the study is concerned with online discourse, not with the participants "as subjects," although I do not ignore the fact that the discourse is produced by "real" people.

Anonymity and informed consent

Most online research contexts follow the Human Subject Model, which prioritizes the protection of privacy of human subjects. The research should not harm the human subject and, therefore, names are to be replaced by pseudonyms, or data should be rendered anonymous. Before the actual start of the empirical research, the researcher needs to obtain informed consent from the subjects involved. But in the realm of Internet research, to blindly apply these ethical rules would result in serious restrictions to the online research. However, contacting the participants regarding informed consent may actually harm the online community involved (King, 1996; Sixsmith and Murray, 2001). For the sake of avoiding obtrusiveness, researchers could choose to remain anonymous themselves. For instance, Smyres (1999) chose not to expose herself as a researcher, because studying teenagers in a natural environment is nearly impossible due to the necessity of parental consent. Bassett and O'Riordan (2002) also argued that it would be a shame if so many of the Internet practices were to remain uninvestigated and opaque if the restraints of the Human Subject Model were always generally applied. Furthermore, seeking informed consent is basically impossible in, for example, the case when a forum is used by a large number of participants or when the participants' contact information is concealed (Döring, 2001). On the other hand, the AoIR states that the greater the participants' vulnerability, the greater is the obligation of the researcher to protect them (Ess and AoIR, 2002).

Seeking informed consent for the analysis of HO-forum threads met serious practical barriers. HO has thousands of participants, who cannot be retrieved because they either hide their email addresses or have long left the forum while their contributions are still accessible in the archive. In these kinds of cases, the AoIR advises considering *whom* to ask for consent – either one asks the administrators or the participants themselves. Thus, I decided to approach the HO's administrators and ask them for consent. Although it is stated in their Rules and Regulations that researchers are not permitted to approach members as research subjects, there seemed to be no problem in contacting the association. After explaining my research interests, the HO association initially balked at my request to approach individual participants because they thought that the researcher's (i.e., my) intrusion would inhibit their participants, which would obviously be inconsistent with the forum's objectives. However, the HO board gave its permission to analyze threads and make quotations from the threads in publications on the condition of anonymity.

Users' nicknames are no longer considered steadfast guarantees of anonymity, as has often been assumed. Registered nicknames are linked to IP addresses, or users may choose to use their own names as nicknames, or they use the same nickname in numerous online environments (Jacobson, 1999). Therefore, the agreement of anonymity was only possible if I agreed not to use the nicknames (and other personal information). Thus, it was not possible to conduct an analysis of nicknames as they occur *in* forum interactions. Another demand that the HO made was that I was not allowed to "follow" single participants, since they wanted to protect individual members from being studied "as subjects." Therefore, the analysis was focused on interaction by many different members and not on single participants' activity or behavior within the involved community.

In recognizing that HO could not give its consent to an analysis of individuals' *nicknames* (obviously these cannot be analyzed anonymously), the participants themselves were asked for permission to have their nicknames included in the data set. HO informed their members on my behalf about the study of the nicknames via a contribution in the forum and requested them to send a reply if they wanted to give their consent. Hence, it became more ethically secure to analyze HO nicknames. However, as a result, the empirical research was presented with two separate data sets: Nicknames and thread conversations. Ethically speaking, the nickname analysis was safer than the thread conversation analyses because of the aforementioned informed consent. I will explain why I did not seek participants' consent for analyzing their forum interactions, because it has been argued that administrators do not have any authority to actually give or deny consent on behalf of their participants (Cherny, 1999). The argument that these discussions take place in a public sphere was also questionable. I will now consider these objections.

In the first place, the HO administrators are more than mere technical providers of a forum; they screen and check contributions, participate in them, edit them when they contain prohibited information and block posters when they do not obey the rules. This suggests that the validity of the administrators' informed consent is very much dependent upon the forum involved and the role of the administrators in that forum. The administrators' active involvement and engagement in HO thus works to justify their claim that informed consent by them may be sufficient.

With regard to the public character of forum communication, Herring (1996) contends that when it is freely available, the interaction is public and thus, in principle, open to research. If the community wishes privacy, private arrangements should be set up and managed, such as Listservs that need the approval of the administrator to join, private chat rooms, etc. However, this argument ignores the fact that *private* interaction is also possible on *public* forums. Moreover, it also fails to recognize that there may be good reasons for not "setting up" technical walls (i.e., registration requirements or permission protocol). In the case of vulnerable or subordinated groups it is extremely important to maintain participation conditions that are as accessible as possible. Similarly, Waskul and Douglas (1996) argued that researchers do not have the right to define which spaces are public and private in order to meet their own research ends. In contrast, other CMC researchers have laid out the public/private distinction in a different way. Paccagnella, for instance, stated:

> We view public discourse on CMC as just that: public. Analysis of such content, where individuals', institutions', and lists' identities are shielded, is not subject to 'Human Subject' restraints. Such study is more akin to the study of tombstone epitaphs, graffiti, or letters to the editor. Personal? – yes. Private? – no (1997: par. 11).

Notwithstanding the attractiveness of adopting this kind of argumentation, conversations can be private for participants in spite of the public setting in which they are held. Therefore, the expectations of the participants are crucial when considering the privacy of online interaction. These expectations are (at least partly) created by the website itself, where the forum is embedded, and also by the actual interactions in the forum. Therefore, the more the public nature is acknowledged, for instance, in its Rules and Regulations regarding participation in the forum, the less obligated one is to protect privacy, confidentiality, the right to informed consent, etc. (see also Ess and AoIR, 2002).

HO, in its Rules and Regulations, which each participant has to agree to before being accepted, announces that postings are saved on the server and that HO takes over joint responsibility for the postings with regard to their public dissemination. Therefore, HO has stated that the participants are also expected to take responsibility for their postings and the disclosure of their real identities (i.e., to register under a valid email address).[35] By mentioning the archiving and by stressing the free and unlimited accessibility of this archive, the forum is presented by HO as more public than private. Furthermore, participants have the ability to shift to private email contact, if they want to avoid the public domain.

To summarize, it appears that HO adequately informs its participants of the public character of the forum and administrators' consent is relatively profound in the case of HO, because moderators are simultaneously active users.

Copyright

The archival characteristic of the Internet renders it a great collection of published texts (Bassett and O'Riordan, 2002). It is not only informed consent that is of interest to the participants, but also the "ownership of their words." In Germany, copyrights legally belong to either (or jointly) the author and/or the publisher of an item of intellectual property (BGBl. I, 2003). When the

[35] Which does not mean that this "real" address has to be publicly visible on the forum; one can choose to hide it.

CMC is seen as the production of discourse or when the participants are regarded as authors, copyright is what counts.[36] However, as soon as the names of "authors" are replaced by pseudonyms, they cannot be given credit for their texts. And it seems that in most Internet research pseudonyms are preferred.

Nevertheless, there is reason to consider copyrights as being relevant to the case of quoting HO-forum contributions. The contributions are publicly available and moreover saved in a freely accessible archive; hence, texts are stored. According to the AoIR, the relevant question is: "Are the participants in this environment best understood as 'subjects' or as authors, whose texts are intended as public?" (2002: 7). In the case of HO, the latter cannot be rejected. Prior to registering, the participant must agree with this aspect of the Rules and Regulations:

> Das Hungrig-Online.de Foren-System arbeitet im Echt-Zeit-Modus. Es ist für das Hungrig-Online-Team daher nicht möglich, die unmittelbare Kontrolle über eingestellte Einträge auszuüben. Wir lesen sehr viele Beiträge, aber nicht alle, und nicht immer sofort. Wir übernehmen keine Verantwortung für den Inhalt, die Richtigkeit und die Form einzelner eingestellter Beiträge. Jeder Verfasser von Einträgen ist als *Autor* selbstverantwortlich für seinen Beitrag. (Emphasis added, W.S.)
>
> (http://www.hungrig-online.de/forum/ubbthreads.php/ubb/newuser)

> [The Hungrig-Online.de System is working in real-time mode. It is impossible for the Hungrig- Online team to have immediate control over posted contributions. We read many of the postings, but not all and not always immediately. We do not take responsibility for the content, the correctness and the form of the individual postings. Each writer of postings is an *author* who is individually responsible for his/her postings.] (Emphasis added, W.S.)

In other words, HO addresses the poster as an author. However, at the bottom of the forum's homepage, HO states that all contributions in the forum fall under the exclusive copyright of the HO association and that they cannot be used, not even when referring to the source. The reason is that media (newspaper, magazines, etc.) may take these postings or quotations out of their

[36] There may be a difference between chat and forum interaction with regard to copyright. Lawson (2004) has suggested that when CMC is ephemeral like speech (which is the case in chats), it is hard to apply copyright law. She called this type of CMC "textoral," neither speech nor text or, to put it differently, a combination of characteristics of speech and text. In the case of bulletin boards or forums, there are less grounds to claim ephemeral speech, since contributions remain on the board and it can take days before a contribution receives a reply.

context and could possibly harm the participants, who may end up reading their own HO postings in a girl's magazine, for instance. Whether this appropriation of copyright is legal or not,[37] it shows that the protection of human subjects, at the same time offering low-threshold accessibility for participants and preventing any unwanted forum quotations from appearing in the popular media are objectives that are apparently hard to secure.

Hybrid ethics

An analysis of the HO forum thus requires an ethical approach that is in congruence with HO's profile and objectives. I do not consider the administrators' informed consent as the only important ethical aspect. I also rely on the arguments that I have collected in this section. First, a critical reading of the HO website revealed that participants are expected to be aware of the public character of their interactions on the forum (the notion of the public forum appears in the Rules and Regulations, the participants are called authors and the postings are stored in the publicly available online archive). Moreover, certain choices in the study of threads more greatly ensure the privacy of the participants. I use pseudonyms for nicknames and modify person-related information, such as geographical location, age, etc. in the thread excerpts. Furthermore, I only used threads from 2005 to avoid postings that have not yet been screened by the administrators. A consequence of using the archive is that many participants who were active in 2005 are no longer active (or are no longer even members) at the time of data collection. If any participant's contact details were available, I have sought to gain consent for the publication of literal quotations (i.e., excerpts) from the author.[38] Explicit consent was received from two members and three moderators; none of the respondents objected to their words being published.

Finally, the reason that the identity of the *website* of HO is not obscured must be explained. HO's priority is to get as much publicity as possible in its attempt to reach those with eating disorders, and, therefore, HO encourages the publication of its Internet address. Any reference to threads or postings in my publications is welcomed, because it directs readers potentially concerned with eating disorders back to HO.[39]

---

[37] I have approached a few German lawyers, but none of them knew for sure if the appropriation of copyright in this case is legal or not.

[38] See Appendix for a copy of the email sent to HO authors.

[39] The additional advantage is that my analyses can be checked in their original setting.

4.4 Data selection and data set

From an ethnomethodological point of view, an indispensable condition for the researchers' attitude during the actual analysis of the data is known as "unmotivated looking," which basically means maintaining one's distance from one's own conventional ideas (Sacks, 1984; Ten Have, 1999). The particular importance of this attitude is that analytical results may differ from what established ideas suggest. In other words, the researcher should not presume or hypothesize, but let the data speak for themselves.[40] As a result, the topic of analysis develops out of the process of analysis. For the present study, this meant starting with an immense source of data: The HO archive. Reading postings and threads from all of the sub-forums since the HO's founding, I early on decided to limit my interest to threads that were archived in early 2005. Here, I found a broad range of interesting phenomena: A wide variety of discussed issues, the apparent avoidance of discussing the "deeper"/psychological causes of participants' eating disorders, the absence of discussions on eating disorders and women, etc. Also, I found the New Here sub-forum especially interesting since its participants actually introduced themselves, which was rarely the case in the other sub-forums. I realized that these threads were particularly sensitive because the new members did not know whether or how they would be accepted by the others. The introductory phase was saliently personal and included numerous expressions of insecurity and hesitancy, which was frequently responded to with expressions of familiarity and solidarity. I asked myself how this level of "closeness" could be explained, because the size of the forum led me to expect a rather anonymous level of participation, which renders "closeness" difficult to develop. This is how I became interested in the phenomenon of entering the forum; it appeared to be not as simple as one may expect from a "low-threshold" online forum. Hence, the topic evolved with more knowledge of the available data, and thus the exact data selection was based on "unmotivated looking" rather than being theory-driven.

As I explained in the previous section, the study is conducted using two separate data sets: A list of nicknames and a set of forum threads. The forum threads were copied from the archive of the New Here sub-forum from 2005. The archive saves threads according to date of last contribution. I chose to use all of the threads from this sub-forum stopping with a contribution that was posted during the first two weeks of 2005. The threads vary in topic, length, number of participants, opening date, etc. But what they have in common is that they all come from the same sub-forum and ended in early

[40] This attitude also resounds in the notion of *ethnomethodological indifference* (Garfinkel and Sacks, 1970, cit. in Ten Have, 1999).

2005. This set contains 37 threads, of which I excluded 10 threads for off-topic reasons: Three are try-out threads by one of the moderators and contained no content, while seven other threads were not related to topic of being a novice in this particular forum. These seven off-topic postings include a personal message from one member to another, a reference to a website, a moderator saying goodbye, a poem, a question about financial support for young people who have left home, complaining about not being able to eat and one report of an intensified eating disorder during a stay abroad. Excluding these threads did not mean they were not interesting (the fact that they were posted in the New Here sub-forum is an interesting finding in itself), but I rejected them because they were not related to the issue of how novice members *enter* the forum. I have not excluded threads opened by non-novice members, who *did* refer to entering HO. Thus, the data set of forum interaction effectively consists of 27 threads, which contain a total of 215 postings, with a great variety of lengths.

One more aspect must be emphasized here. It is a participant's personal choice whether s/he contributes to the New Here sub-forum, which means that it is very likely that the members end up circumventing the New Here sub-forum and immediately participate in other sub-forums.

The data collection of nicknames is described in chapter 5.

4.5 Methods of analysis

An interaction analysis as empirical method can reveal certain aspects of a phenomenon, but not all of them. The present study applies an interaction analysis based on discourse analysis and specifically CA to investigate the interactive (i.e., constituted in turns) process of entering an online community, including, for instance, the thresholds that novices may encounter or regular members may create. In the first place, an interaction analysis reveals how participants of a particular discussion or a thread of postings among themselves negotiate meanings. This implies that (semantic) relations are constructed or attended to in the discourse itself. The action orientation of an utterance (i.e., what an utterance "does") is mainly the result of the relations between the utterances of the larger stretch of discourse. Moreover, referential utterances do not only derive their meaning from the world outside of the discourse, but also from other parts of the same discourse. This view and focus is programmatic for conversation analysis and, in fact, a consequent continuation of the project of ethnomethodology (Weeks, 1995).

However, an interaction analysis also sheds light on the connection of the micro- and macro-levels of discourse. Therefore, it is related to other types of discourse analysis, which I will explain in the next sub-section. Both discourse-analytical dimensions ranging from micro-/text-based to macro-level form the epistemological basis of this analysis.

Discourse Analysis

The object of analysis of the current study can be described as discourse, which means that I take the HO interactions and nicknames as language used in context. On the one hand, this view of language must be distinguished from traditional linguistics, where language is merely viewed as a system in itself.[41] On the other hand, I do not use the concept of discourse in the Foucauldian sense of an individualizable group of statements, such as the discourse of femininity or the discourse of imperialism (Mills, 2004: 6), which is an abstract notion of discourse related to clusters of ideas rather than the object of an empirical analysis. Following Jaworski and Coupland, I understand discourse as

> language use relative to social, political and cultural formations – it is language reflecting social order but also language shaping social order, and shaping individuals' interaction with society (1999: 3).

The various approaches of discourse analysis rely on different concepts of discourse. Generally, I understand the "task" of discourse analysis as "to show how micro-level social actions realize and give local form to macro-level social structures" (Jaworski and Coupland, 1999: 12). This means that my analysis is a micro-level study of language-in-use under the assumption that macro-level phenomena can, and should be studied on the level of real people's lives, which takes place partly in or through language. Jaworski and Coupland (1999: 12-13) mention various aspects that such an analysis should attend to, of which I would like to mention four.

> 1. The meaning of an event or of a single utterance is only partly accounted for by its formal features (that is, by the 'direct meaning' of the words used). The social significance of discourse, if we define it simply as language in use, lies in the relationship between linguistic meanings and the wider context (i.e. the social, cultural, economic, demographic and other characteristics of the communicative event) in which the interaction takes place (1999: 12).

---

[41] Benveniste (1971: 110, cited in Mills, 1997: 4) emphasized this distinction from "language as a system" as follows: "The sentence, an undefined creation of limitless variety, is the very life of human speech in action. We conclude from this that with the sentence we leave the domain of language as a system of signs and enter into another universe, that of language as an instrument of communication, whose expression is discourse."

I have mentioned that the "wider context" of the HO forum can be seen as a Community of Practice, but it is also characterized by socio-medical structures in the field of eating disorders, such as diagnostic criteria, statistics on eating disorders and the phenomenon of the pro-eating disorders movement.

> 2. Our interpretation of discourse [...] relates far more to what is done by participants than what is said (or written, or drawn, or pointed at) by them. That is, a functional analysis of language and other semiotic systems lies at the heart of analyzing discourse (1999: 13).

This point reflects, or explains the ethnomethodological perspective I have taken with regard to both identity and community. I focus on what participants *do* or accomplish with what they have written in their HO postings, rather than on the content of their postings as such.

> 3. It is important to distinguish between meanings (including goals and intentions) inferred by observers and meanings (including goals and intentions) inferred by participants. Analyzing discourse is often making inferences about inferences. (1999: 13).

My interpretation of discursive actions is not necessarily a reflection or representation of the meaning that HO participants (would claim to) attach to their actions. My interpretations are connected to observable discourse features within postings, and in the sequences of postings. Thereby, they become analyses, which are again "tested" on how participants deal with them. Still, in spite of the focus on participants' orientations, how I phrase my analyses inevitably offers inferences regarding what the participants actually did.

> 4. Discourse analysis provides a way of linking up the analysis of local characteristics of communication to the analysis of broader social characteristics. It can let us see how macro-structures are carried out through micro-structures (1999: 13).

By sketching the socio-medical picture of eating disorders (chapter 3), I intended to provide a macro-level overview as the societal background of the micro-level analysis. I have methodically attempted to not presume that "given" macro-structures are acted out on the micro-level, but to instead be attentive to a relation between the macro- and micro-levels, which does not mean that participants are principally unable to resist certain macro-structures. Thus, I avoided considering participants as cultural dopes (cf. Garfinkel, 1967).

Conversation Analysis

The study of forum interactions requires a method of analyzing discourse, which is, in the first place, sensitive to interaction as a specific type of discourse, and secondly, compatible with the ethnomethodological premise of accomplishing things with/through language. For this reason, I have applied the perspective and the concepts of conversation analysis (CA). CA originates from, and therefore is related to other sociological theories.

From Goffman, it has adopted the assumption that talk-in-interaction is a fundamental social domain that can be examined as an institutional entity in its own right and from Garfinkel, it took the notion that practices and procedures with which parties produce and recognize that talk are actually talk's *ethnomethods* (Heritage, 2001).

CA was initiated by Harvey Sacks and further developed by Emanuel Schegloff and Gail Jefferson. Generally put, it investigates what methods individuals employ to make sense of their world, how they display this understanding to others, and how they produce the mutually shared social order in which they live (Drew, 2005). Discursive psychologists, who use a very similar instrumentarium as conversation analysts, have emphasized the fundamentally social aspect of these processes in opposition to a psychological or cognitive character (e.g., Edwards, 1997; Edwards and Potter, 1992; Potter, 1996; Potter and Wetherell, 1987). Participants' sensitivity to positions, accounts and dilemmas as it is displayed in talk is not seen as a representation of a mental state (Edwards, 1997). Rather, interactional accomplishments are viewed as stemming from individuals that have an *interest* in presenting the world in one way rather than in another. And this is oriented to in the turn-by-turn conduct of conversation. In line with this, CA avoids offering descriptions of social settings that compete with the actual descriptions produced by the individuals who are party to those settings. Put differently, CA seeks to describe the conversational methods that individuals themselves use in their actual descriptions of settings. Hence, it analyzes *how* people do things, rather than *why* they do them. CA work conducted thus far has already yielded a great body of knowledge on how conversation works, concentrating on turns, turn design, sequence (organization) and intersubjectivity (Drew, 2005). For the actual analysis, this knowledge (for example, the groundbreaking research on adjacency pairs [Schegloff, 1968] and preference [Pomerantz, 1984] is used and applied).

Concretely, three assumptions inform conversation analysis (Heritage, 2001). First, sequential positioning is considered as a resource for the production and understanding of utterances (Schegloff, 1984). It classically focuses on the question: Why do we find this utterance here? (Schegloff, 1997). A second aspect is the projection of relevance. This means that current actions ordinarily project the relevance of next actions to be done by a subsequent speaker. For instance, questions project the relevance of answers, or greetings the relevance of return greetings. These kinds of pairs are called adjacency pairs, which are a powerful device in interactions, which can be observed when, for instance, a question does not elicit a response. This *noticeable absence* (Schegloff, 1968) underlines the normativity of certain patterns of interaction. The third assumption follows from the second: The next action of a subsequent speaker shows an understanding of a prior action. So, an answer is a display of the understanding of the previous turn as a question. The absence of an answer can accordingly be interpreted as not having understood the utterance as a question, which may lead the speaker to repeat or reformulate the question (cf. Hutchby and Wooffitt, 1998: 42).

Traditionally, CA involves the collection and transcription of audio or audio-visual recordings of conversation, but it has also been proposed for the analysis of computer-mediated communication (e.g., Herring, 2004). The methodology of CA cannot be transferred one-to-one to computer-mediated conversation: Turns and turn design are different because overlap, interruption and phonetic marking are impossible in typed CMC. However, other conversation analytical focal points can be adopted: The sequential organization, the global organization (of postings), and demonstrations of interpretation in assessments and formulations. In other words, in computer-mediated interaction language can also be studied for how it is used to perform actions in the specific online setting in connection to the sequential organization of the interaction. This means that to understand which action is being done depends not only on the broader social setting, but particularly on what has been said or typed before, and after. CA assumes that it is not only researchers who can observe this, but that crucially, members (i.e., the interactants) are sensitive to the actions being performed in their encounters, and that they may articulate their understanding of them in a subsequent turn.[42] For instance, in an online forum interaction we may also find accounts. Accounts are descriptions that "name, characterize, formulate, explain, excuse, excoriate, or merely take notice of some circumstance or activity and thus place it within some social framework" (West and Zimmerman, 1987: 136). Focusing on turns in interaction, accountability thus refers to how "actors design their actions in relation to their circumstances so as to permit others, by methodically taking account of circumstances, to recognize the action for what it is" (Heritage, 1984: 179).

Also identity (Benwell and Stokoe, 2006; Schegloff, 2007; Zimmerman, 1998) can be analyzed in CMC data and even easier than in spoken data in

[42] Participants' sensitivity may not be misunderstood as participants' awareness or intentionality; conversation analysts and discursive psychologists prefer to remain agnostic on this issue (e.g., Potter, 1996). Put differently, CA is not interested in mental or cognitive states, but in the norms that are operative in the conduct of action, in how people do things in talk (Drew, 2005).

which demonstrable relevance is more difficult to determine. Demonstrable relevance of social identities in talk has led to heated debates about CA (Billig, 1999a, 1999b; Schegloff, 1997, 1999a, 1999b; Wetherell, 1998), and so I chose to analyze clearly demonstrable identities in my data. For CMC, demonstrability depends on visibility rather than audibility. As a consequence, a conversation analysis of CMC does not require transcription. Furthermore, pitch and voice, which frequently display gender (as an identity), are lacking. Moreover, in the forum names and membership positions are visible for any contribution, equally for members and analysts. As a result, the relevance of identities is observable both for members and analysts in what is readable on the computer's screen. Hence, although a pure CA study of CMC is impossible, because CMC lacks many features of spoken interaction, an "applied" form of CA is useful for the analysis of CMC.

To summarize, I use CA concepts as the methodological instrumentation for an analysis of online interaction. The analytical focal points are, on the one hand, the global and sequential organization of forum postings and threads and, on the other hand, identities, accounts and assessments. The analysis of nicknames differs in orientation, since the ethical concern has rendered it unfavorable to approach them in their sequential appearance. In chapter 5, I describe how I proceeded with this part of the study.

Analytical procedure

I have conducted sequence analyses of the 27 threads. The comparability of threads enabled by the data set was taken advantage of here. The 27 forum threads made it possible to observe regularities and therefore also so-called "deviant cases." These cases worked to reinforce the analysis, since they showed participants' orientation both toward the normative requirements and the excusability or local rationality of deviance from it (Ten Have, 1999: 137). In the present study, this type of comparison was procedurally exploited, because the sequence analysis of the threads yielded the observation that some threads seemed to be similar, whereas a few were notably different. This kind of sequence analysis was conducted predominantly by me, but additionally in data sessions with fellow researchers. This helped to establish the fact that my interpretation was not particularistic. For the presentation of the findings, I adopted the extremely useful feature of discourse research to quote the original data, which enables the reader to make her/his own judgments about the researcher's interpretations.

Moreover, I have considered the data in relation to, and for its coherence with previous work in the field of ethnomethodology and CA. In chapters 6 through 8 I explicitly quote these studies to establish the analysis of the HO-forum interaction in this broader empirical arena, and to bring to light salient similarities and differences.

This analytic procedure clarified various topics of interest. It was observed that many of the threads started with a highly hesitant and uncertain utterance and that many responses to these kinds of postings offered warm welcomes. This is examined in detail in chapter 6. Second, it was striking that in some threads, the novice member appeared to be rather ignorant about the nature of her/his eating disorder. I wondered whether the HO forum was not being used as an *alternative* to medical consultation, but used for the posing of diagnostic questions. However, on a second occasion, I realized that these were actually just exceptions. Most novice participants introduced themselves as clearly eating disordered, namely through diagnoses of eating disorders. Notably, age and the duration of one's eating disorder also continued to return time and again in these self-presentations. Congruently, chapter 7 investigates self-presentations and ways that recipients deal with them in the HO forum, which is explained by the relevance of accountability. The exceptional cases showed the normativity of these regular cases. After a close analysis of these, I decided to devote a chapter (8) to two exemplary "deviant" cases. Thus, the analytical procedure of finding regularities and exceptions is reflected in the composition of the research findings; chapter 6 and 7 focus more on regularities, whereas chapter 8 highlights "deviant" cases.

The analysis of nicknames was conducted as a supplement to the interaction analysis, as an acknowledgement of the fact that they characterize their referents in various ways, among which gender. I did not collect any personal information from the HO participants, which means that their nicknames are frequently the only means to somehow establish a portrait of who is actually posting at HO.

Chapter 5

Identity accomplished through nicknames

5.1 Introduction

Becoming a member of HO requires a unique nickname, which makes nicknames crucial entities in the process of entering the forum. With the first visit to the forum it quickly becomes clear that HO nicknames are funny, telling or strange, which means that they are not irrelevant labels. Some nicknames seem "typically" feminine, whereas others seem to express strength, some are incomprehensible, and some are "just" popular first names. Compare *lillifee79*, *Kassiopaiah, Sophia_21, marienblume* (German "daisy") and *quorkepf*, probably from *Querkopf* (German "awkward customer"). Some nicknames clearly give the impression that the member is female, whereas others appear more neutral at first sight. Participants with more or less "gender neutral" nicknames do not introduce themselves as "woman"/"girl" or "man"/"boy," which implies that *if* gender is displayed at all, it is usually through nicknames. These two initial impressions (nicknames are telling and can convey gender) have resulted in the decision to analyze nicknames in how they accomplish identity attributes more generally and gender in particular. I will now explain this in a little more detail.

The first impetus for the analysis is the inventiveness and eye-catching nature of many of the nicknames, but also the value members claim to attach to them. In forum threads, participants reflect upon their meanings and explain the personal or emotional value of their nicknames. An exploratory look into various sub-forums of the HO forum reveals a great interest in the power of nicknames as self-constructing units. Five (translated) utterances (drawn from the HO forum but not from the data set) illustrate this.

1. If I changed my nickname, it would feel as if I was giving up a part of myself.
2. Mein Nick bin ich ('my nick is me'), I would never change it!

Utterance (1) underlines the importance of a nickname to the self, as if losing the nickname would be like losing an arm. Even if "part" is meant metaphorically, it still suggests that the nickname is treated as an essential component of the self. Example (2) is even more striking; it declares that the nickname is identical to the self. This one-to-one mapping of nickname with self seems positive, in terms of accepting the nickname as one is supposed to accept oneself. It implies that changing one's nickname would affect the self. The following quotes further illustrate the relationship between the nickname and the self:

3. When I feel well, I am irritated by my nick, but apart from that, it fits.
4. If I get better at some point, I will need a new nick…

In (3) it appears that the nickname stands for the negative state of the self. First, it is presupposed that the "I" knows two conditions: Feeling well and one that is "apart from" feeling well. The nickname fits the latter condition and is thereby a constituent of the negative self. A similar interpretation can be read from (4), where the nickname is temporarily bound to the current state of the self, namely the eating disordered self. The final example (5) shows how the nickname can become more important than one's actual first name, implying that the nickname does its job of constructing identity better than someone's first name:

5. I identify more with [nickname], than with my real name.

The analysis presented below reveals the types of names that fulfill this essential task.

The second impetus is the question of gender. In the data set of 27 threads, I found only one male participant (i.e., a member who somehow presented himself as a man). His nickname is not obviously male or female. However, this member began his first posting by giving his "real" first name, a commonly known male name in Germany. Consider the opening of his posting.

Excerpt 1 (#A20)
[Nickname]*: Hallo und ein Frohes neues!
hallo
ich möchte mich auch noch mal kurz vorstellen,
also ich heiße [a commonly known male first name]* und ich komme aus [city in Germany]*
naja ich bin jetzt auch schon seit einiger zeit mit ES am kämpfen und immerwider pleiten erlebt [*sic*].

[Nickname]: Hello and a Happy New Year!
hello

i would also like to briefly introduce myself briefly,
*so my name is [a commonly known male first name] and i come from [city in Germany]**
well, i've been fighting with ED for some time now and have experienced failure over and over again.

* The names in this posting are deleted for ethical reasons (see 4.3).

The 27 threads I analyzed do not comprise enough material to conclude that *only* male novice members offer their gendered "real" name in their self-presentations. There is also no indication that co-participants somehow "orient to" this unexpected gender (i.e., none of the respondents to the posting in excerpt 1 somehow react to the fact that this member is male). This seems unusual, since, in previous research, cases of recipient orientation to the (unexpected) gendered name *have* been found. For instance, Wilkinson and Kitzinger (2007) analyzed a call in which a female caller explicitly refers to her partner (a woman) by using her partner's name, after the call-taker had demonstrated to assume that the partner is a man. Hence, the "unexpected" gender is thus *locally* oriented to by saying a name. In the excerpt above, it is the less local context – namely other first postings – that makes this male name more salient. From this perspective, the fact that other novice members (the others in the data set all seem to be female, which is based either on their nicknames, pronouns, stereotypical female activities, or heterosexual relationships) do not "produce" their real first name to present their gender as notable.[43] Usually, only nicknames exhibit participants' gender, if at all. Hence, it appears that names may be important for the articulation of gender.

Before I turn to the analysis of HO nicknames, I will first consider a theoretical understanding of nicknames in relation to identity. In studies of discourse it is common to draw on concepts from both the social sciences and linguistics. The first discipline interrogates the social relevance of the use of names in social life, whereas a linguistic analysis is useful for an understanding of what types of names are used and what cultural associations are invoked by them. In this chapter, earlier research on names in relation to community is touched upon. Subsequently, I elaborate on the concept of nicknames as actor-focal emblems (Agha, 2007) which will lead to an approach that analyzes

---

[43] A potential explanation for the rare occurrence of "doing" gender other than through a nickname (for instance, saying that you are a girl) is that participants presuppose that their fellow members are female, which renders it unnecessary to make gender relevant at the point of entering the forum. Thus, it would also explain that in excerpt 1, a male participant "does" gender particularly clearly at the beginning of his posting.

nicknames connected to members' identities. Subsequently, the link between gender and names will be examined more closely.

5.2 Theorizing names sociologically and linguistically

I will first briefly consider the role that names can play in a community from a sociological viewpoint. Chapter 2 already noted that when a newcomer enters a so-called total institution s/he may be given a new name by the inmates as a way of stripping the newcomer of her/his social identity, which is typical for this kind of community (Goffman, 1961). In online forums, it is not the "inmates" who enforce this nickname upon the newcomer, but the novice her/himself who carries out this self-constitutive act. It is not the aim of this study to interrogate why or how members choose the names they do, but rather to conduct an analysis that presumes that names in a specific context bring forth a world of cultural associations. According to Rymes, names fulfill all kinds of social functions in addition to referring to a specific situation: "Names serve to describe individual traits; they index familiarity, kinship and group membership; they pick out entire worlds of cultural significance" (1996: 242). The fact that someone can have different names in different communities suggests a connection between the community and the name. Looking at a specific community, members' local names may thus be taken to reflect community membership.

In transferring these aspects of names to the present study, it must be emphasized that HO is a *peer community*, and not a public medium that is directed at a potentially larger or broader audience (such as blogs, websites as well as advertisements). This means that the term cultural representation or cultural significance must be used with caution. Part of the cultural significance of names is that names are cultural representations (cf. Engel, 2002; Hall, 1997).[44] In the analysis of representations, analysts frequently use material such as advertisements. It is assumed that particular forms of difference or "Otherness" (Hall, 1997) are constructed in advertisements. Viewing eating disorders as a stigma highlights their social deviance with respect to the society or culture at large or compared to "normals" (Goffman, 1986). The cultural representation conveyed through nicknames in the HO forum should not, however, be confused with that of advertisements. Despite the fact that the forum is publicly accessible, we should not assume that they are primarily representations aimed at a general public. They should be considered the participants' constructions in/for the HO community instead. Although, in the present analysis, they are read as cultural representations, I do recognize their

[44] According to Engel (2002: 18), representation is a social practice or technology that works constitutively, which means that it produces meaning and constructs reality.

occurrence in places like the HO community in particular. Despite the fact that links are sought between (studies on) eating disorders and the nicknames as cultural representations, suggestions of causal or intentional links are avoided. If it had been at all possible to contact HO members, then another interpretation more closely related to the community, could have been added, but as it is explained in section 4.3, this was not a reasonable option.

The present analysis serves to describe how HO nicknames construct character traits possibly related to eating disorders (not because members may *have* an eating disorder, but because they use the nickname *in a forum on eating disorders*). The shortcoming of the analysis is that the nicknames cannot be studied for how they are embedded in surrounding talk. In other words, their referential work and their context-bound use in this specific forum remain unexplored. Therefore, the analysis cannot conclude anything about the actual use of names in the HO forum. However, it can interpret their cultural significance, including the personal traits that are invoked by them, and thus reveal at least something about who is posting in HO.

Linguistically, nicknames are proper names. A characteristic of proper names is that their reference, unlike the reference of pronouns and demonstratives, does not shift from speech event to speech event (also called *speech-chain deictics*). In other words, what makes a proper name special is that it has an identical referent on different occasions. In addition to indicating a unique referent, a proper name can also have a denotation. Traditionally, denotation in contrast to reference is considered utterance independent (J. Lyons, 1995). For example, phrases like *my dog*, *the dog*, and *the dog that bit the postman* have different referents but the same denotation, to the extent that they are all members of the class *dogs*. However, this is only true in the case of literal usage; a metaphorical use of *dog* does not denote a member of the class dogs (Agha, 2007), for instance *dirty dog*. Therefore, denotation is also event dependent, although not in the same way as reference. These differences in denotation and reference can be schematically summarized as in table 1.

	Denotation	Reference
Noun phrases (e.g., the dog, my dog)	Event independent	Event dependent
Noun phrases – metaphorical (e.g., dirty dog)	Event dependent	Event dependent
Proper names (e.g., nicknames)	(Partly) event dependent	Event independent

Table 1. Denotation and reference of noun phrases, metaphorical noun phrases and proper names.

In the present study, the focus is on nicknames as denotational units in a specific event and as actor-focal emblems, which means that they hold identity-ascribing features (Agha, 2007). The actor-focal dimension in nicknames has been neglected in previous research on nicknames, in which only denotations (or literal meanings) were distinguished (cf. Bechar-Israeli, 1995).

As an alternative to the term *identity*, which itself does not focus on the processes by which identity is formed, Agha proposes the concept of *emblem*. An emblem involves three elements: 1) a perceivable thing/a diacritic, 2) a social persona, and 3) someone for whom it is an emblem. The focus needs to be on the relation between these elements – that is to say, not on the "thing" or on persona alone, but on acts or performances through which the two are linked. Emblems accomplish various types of identity. One type of emblem is the registered[45] emblem, through which people can be allocated registered identities, such as female, upper class, and lawyer. (In chapter 2, this type of identity was labeled *categorical identity*). Nicknames as actor-focal emblems can thus be read for how they convey such social identity categories, but they also enact person attributes, or personal identity. Emblems can construct personal identity through stereotypic images. Nevertheless, the fact that a decontextualized analysis of stereotypes was short term I already noted in chapter 2. The event of occurrence of HO nicknames (i.e., a German forum on eating disorders) needs to be taken into account when analyzing HO nicknames and their emblematic person attributes. Hence, Agha's theory of language and social relations allows for an understanding of nicknames textualized in a specific event as proper names, which can have denotational, event-dependent properties, but also as actor-focal emblems, which construe attributes of the actor who performs the signs partly by means of stereotypes. In the next section, I will specify the methodological steps I took for this type of analysis, but first I will specify the ways in which gender can

[45] For an explanation of the concept of *register*, see Agha (2007, chapters 2 and 3).

be constructed in nicknames namely both through denotation and through stereotypes.

Doing gender through nicknames

In section 5.1, the expectation that gender could be accomplished through nicknames was related to a perspective on nicknames as entities that *possibly* "do" a gender category (female/male). Although nicknames are frequently regarded for their gender potential in studies on online communication, this is operationalized more as a means to determine the participants' gender, than investigated as a topic in itself. Moreover, the way in which semantic criteria apply in gender determination is not specified in these studies. For instance, the Thai nickname *Maunjalho* is classified as male because it means "seems smart" and *Maunsuey* is classified as female, because it means "seems beautiful" (Panyametheekul and Herring, 2003: n.p.). In the present study, gender is not analyzed in order to determine the participants' gender, but to understand if and how it is conveyed as a person attribute (and thus as an identity) in nicknames of the HO forum. For this reason, the present study focuses on the features that render a nickname gendered (or not). Thus, the nickname *Maunsuey* ("seems beautiful"), which denotes the feature "beautiful," and is stereotypically read as feminine, would be analyzed as an actor-focal emblem of femininity.

Gender is an identity category in names that can be conveyed both through denotation and stereotypic effects. I will explain this in more detail. First of all, gender can often be identified in the phonological and morphological features of names. In German, names ending in *-a* or *-e* are almost always female, and names ending in *-n*, *-s* or *-d* are predominantly male (Gerhards, 2003). Not surprisingly, nicknames in the HO forum display these "gendered" phonological features. Especially in nicknames that are novel formations (i.e., they possess no lexical denotation), the phonological features may make the nickname seem female or male. In this way, for example, the nickname *kareja* seems female, because of the ending *-a*.

A different type of nickname, consisting of a personal noun or noun phrase such as *Blue Guy*, constructs gender through the lexical gender of the personal noun (Hellinger and Bußmann, 2001). Hence, the nickname *Blue Guy* denotes a male. In such cases, gender is very apparent in the nickname. *Apparent* gender has been characterized as typical for online communication (Herring, 2001), but in the HO forum there are many nicknames that are less or seemingly not gendered. However, if nicknames are viewed as emblems, the stereotypic effects of nicknames in text-in-context can still be related to gender. For instance, nicknames in the HO forum that denote flowers metaphorically index femininity, such as *marienblume* (German "daisy"). The actor-focal emblem *marienblume* constructs the actor, i.e., this particular HO participant, as sweet, small, and innocent (see also section 5.5 below).

Hence, gender in nicknames can be read in phonological/morphological, denotational and stereotypical features. However, these features can also work reciprocally. For example, the grammatical gender of nouns may be related to the ascription of stereotypically gendered attributes to the actor. Konishi (1991) showed that high frequency words in German carry connotations of femininity and masculinity, depending on their grammatical gender. For instance, the nickname **Schneeflocke** (German "snowflake") is grammatically feminine and may also be read as stereotypically feminine because of its attributes of softness, lightness, etc. This happens in other grammatical gender languages as well. A nickname such as *tortuga* (Spanish "turtle"), which is grammatically feminine, may also be stereotypically feminine. Put differently, a reading of turtle as an emblem constructs attributes such as small, peaceful, and reliable.[46] These characteristics are stereotypically feminine, which corresponds with *tortuga*'s grammatical gender.

Method

As indicated earlier, I used a pragmatic approach (in the linguistic sense) for the analysis of nicknames, which links denotation and stereotypes to the indexical context of the nicknames, which are the participants of the HO forum. This means that a nickname discursively constructs personal attributes of the indexed participant through its denotation and stereotypical features (see 2.7 for the link between nicknames and personal identity). The analysis of nicknames started by determining for each nickname its denotational properties and its emblematic (actor-focal, context-bound) stereotypical person attributes including gender (Agha, 2007). For the reading of nicknames as emblems – a concept in which the person who reads the signs is explicitly incorporated – I was the main reader of the nicknames in this study. Additionally, mother tongue speakers of German and research colleagues were asked to contribute their readings and understandings of the nicknames. Thereafter, commonalities and differences among the nicknames were grouped, first, with respect to denotational properties and, second, on the level of actor-focal emblems for various person attributes.

For reading denotations, a distinction was made between the literal and metaphorical use in relation to the event (the HO forum). HO nicknames denoting a plant, an animal, or a star were read metaphorically. Moreover, a nickname that denotes "child" was read metaphorically in HO (i.e., not liter-

---

[46] These associations could be related to the "babyness" of small animals (Lorenz, 1943), which means that humans perceive small animals that share certain physical features with human babies (such as large head and eyes) as cute and sweet.

ally denoting a child, but a person who is like a child). Similarly, the nickname *Pueppi23*, which denotes "small doll" in certain settings, where the referent is a member of the class *dolls*, should be read metaphorically as a silly, over-dressed woman in HO.

5.3 Data

The set of nicknames forms a different kind of discourse than the set of interactions, due to the ethical concern of hiding personal information (see 4.3).

Data collection

The data set of nicknames was collected in cooperation with HO. The HO team manager introduced the research to the forum and asked for consent to allow the analysis of participants' nicknames. The manager's request mentioned that a linguistic analysis of the nicknames was the focus of the research. Furthermore, participants were discouraged from giving consent if they felt that their nickname divulged personal information (for example, if they also used the same nickname in other web-based environments). The request was posted in early August 2006. After three weeks, a total of 83 participants had given their consent by directly and publicly replying to the manager's request.[47] The participants also posed many questions and gave encouraging comments, which underscores that the participants themselves had a sincere interest or curiosity in (an analysis of) their nicknames.[48]

[47] A limitation of this part of the study is therefore the relatively small number of nicknames used for analysis. Furthermore, the method of data collection, although ethically sound, is problematic. For example, a call for participation and consent may be answered by those who are particularly proud of their nicknames, resulting in a biased sample.

[48] Furthermore, after the publication of the analysis of nicknames in the Journal of Computer-Mediated Communication (Stommel, 2007), I asked the HO contact person whether he would be willing to inform HO members about the study. He did so by placing a hyperlink to the article in the forum. This led to a generally positive chain reaction. Some HO members (among whom were a few linguists) took the initiative to work on a German translation of the article, at least of the main findings, to make the article more accessible to German readers. I have still not been informed about the progress of this initiative to this very day, but it does underscore the interest of HO members in their community and willingness to contribute to it.

Data

The nickname corpus consists of various word and phrase types, as summarized in table 2. The analysis first distinguishes between names (= proper nouns) and nouns (= common nouns).[49] Names are further sub-divided into commonly known names and novel formations. Nouns are sub-divided into personal nouns (i.e., nouns which denote people) and other nouns.[50]

Word and phrase types in HO nicknames	Number of nicknames
Commonly known names	
a) first names	34
b) place names	2
Novel formations (e.g., *kareja, Lupasimo, Nezadim*)	7
Nouns and noun phrases	
a) personal nouns (e.g., *Ampelweibchen* – German "small traffic light female," *Ms. Dust, Blue Guy*)	8
b) other nouns (e.g., *baerli* – German "small bear," *snjor-blom* – Icelandic "snow flower")	25
Adjectives (e.g., *nice*)	3
Verb forms (e.g., **Vivo** – Italian "I live")	2
Exclamations (e.g., *nixwieweg* – German "let's get out of here")	2
TOTAL	**83**

Table 2. Word and phrase types in the corpus of HO nicknames

[49] The reason for not using the grammatical terms "proper nouns" vs. "common nouns" is that, in fact, all nicknames are proper nouns. However, a distinction needs to be made between nicknames that are already known as names (commonly known names), and nicknames that are either possible but unattested names (novel formations) or are made up of nouns or other linguistic forms (other word types such as verbs, adjectives and exclamations).

[50] In the HO forum, the name of a famous person does not refer to that famous person in particular, but to a HO member. As a consequence, the name must be seen as an emblem, intended to be read as such by other forum participants. In this way, stereotypical attributes of the famous referent are projected onto the HO participant.

The goal of the analysis of the nicknames found on the HO forum is to examine if and how participants accomplish identity (including gender) through nicknames, and to explore potential relationships to the various eating disorders.

5.4 Analysis: Female names and a great variety of language origins

Almost half of the set of 83 nicknames are more or less common first names, such as *Samirah* and *Ivon*. The corpus includes 34 first names, of which 25 are female, seven male, and two that could be either female or male. In the group of other nouns, gender plays an evident role. Of the eight personal nouns in the forum, five are lexically female, one lexically male, and two are not lexically gendered. Of the other nouns (25), 11 appeared to be grammatically feminine, two masculine, and eight neuter. Taken together, the first names and nouns (67 of the total of 83 nicknames = 81 %) show a clear predominance of femaleness. However, the nicknames are not always gendered. For instance, the nickname *paper cup* does not seem to be gendered in the HO context. Therefore, although gender seems to be an important identity category in HO nicknames, it is not obligatory.

Language origin

The nicknames show a rich variety of language origins. The languages used, including the languages from which the commonly known first names are derived, are: German, Southern German, Spanish, English, Italian, Swedish, Icelandic, Latin, Turkish, Greek, Arabic, Bulgarian, Chinese, Finnish, Hungarian, and Czech. In terms of identity, the participants with non-German nicknames (which are not commonly used in German contexts) seem special, distinctive, or even exotic.

Many nicknames that are first names are of non-German origin. *Iveta* is a Czech first name, *Raya* is Bulgarian, *Alessia* is Italian, and *Finja* is Finnish. Modifications appear in spelling or in the addition of numbers, such as in *Sophia_21*. These first names are coded for gender, which means that they are stereotypical indexicals for females or males. Another set of nicknames is not gender coded. They seem to be novel formations, i.e., newly invented. Only their phonological endings make them sound like female or male names, e.g., *kareja* and *Taurelia*. These endings render the nicknames gendered and thus attribute gender as a durable characteristic to the person carrying the nickname.

5.5 Analysis denotations: Natural, small, light, derogatory or noble

The group of nicknames that are not commonly known or popular proper names reveal several denotational patterns. As shown in table 3, flora, fauna, and meteorology/astrology, as various aspects of nature, are common lexical resources for HO nicknames. It can generally be argued that in occidental culture, nature (when not conceived of as aggressive, wild, or powerful, but rather as "mother earth") is linked to femininity, which renders a "nature" nickname a demeanor indexical of a specific type of femininity. However, such meanings are highly dependent on the specific context. More precisely, the meaning of a metaphor such as "woman is nature" is dependent on where, in which Community of Practice, it occurs (Eckert and McConnell-Ginet, 2003). In the HO forum, with its very high percentage of young women struggling with eating disorders, even in nicknames such as *Loewen_maeulchen* (German "small snap dragon," but also "small lion's mouth") and *baerli* (German "small bear"), the "smallness" of the animals involved suggests that they should not be read as aggressive, masculine manifestations of nature. A small bear is a cuddly toy rather than an aggressive beast.

Flora	Fauna	Meteorology/astrology
Loewen_maeulchen (German "small snap dragon")	Song_bird	Lluvia (Spanish "rain")
Snjorblum (Icelandic "snow flower")	Schattenvoegelchen (German "small shadow bird")	*Schneeflocke* (German "snowflake")
blackroseGeb1987 (Geb = geboren – German "born")	baerli (German "small bear")	Cielo (Italian/Spanish "sky"/"heaven")
marienblume (German "daisy")	tortuga (Spanish "turtle")	Estrella1981 (Spanish "star")

Table 3. Examples of nicknames in the category "nature"

In addition to being related to nature, these nicknames denote other interesting aspects. Most nicknames in the "nature" category denote *small* animals, flowers, or plants. "Smallness" or diminutiveness (e.g., by using diminutive suffixes in German) can be considered a metaphorical property of femaleness on the grounds that women are typically physically smaller than men, but also (and more interestingly) because it treats women like children, small animals, and other things that are harmless, vulnerable, and cute. This cultural representation of femininity has been identified by, amongst others, second-wave feminists (Beauvoir, 1992/1949; Friedan, 1966/1963; Millett, 1985/1969). Moreover, "small" maps metaphorically onto "insignificant," "trivial," and "less important." Smallness in nicknames as applied to the self could thus be interpreted as signaling femaleness, child-like qualities, and/or self-deprecation. Smallness together with childishness may have a special meaning for those with eating disorders, namely as the opposite of fat. Orbach explains the relation between fat, need and smallness:

> Fat has come to stand for need, greed, indulgence, wantonness, unruliness, a loss of control, an unstoppability. Fatness represents folds and folds of uncontrollable needs and the guilt associated with the satisfaction of such needs. Fat represents the *exposure* of need. The ability to make herself smaller and smaller is the direct expression of the anorectic's success in controlling such needs and neediness (2001: 91 emphasis in original).

Another observation is that almost all of these nicknames denote light or weightless things or beings, such as rain, snow, stars, and sky, but also small animals and flowers. The nicknames which denote lightness or weightlessness are congruent with the anorectic's and bulimic's fear of taking up space in the world and the ideal of thinness or even weightlessness (Bruch, 2001). Bigness, fatness, and heaviness do not appear in the nicknames.[51] Orbach (2001) notes that as the body has come to represent the existence and insistence of needs, the anorectic develops the wish to do away with the body or exist without a body at all. Nicknames such as *Estrella1981* (Spanish "star"), *cielo* (Italian/Spanish "sky"/"heaven"), **Schneeflocke** (German "snowflake"), and *Lluvia* (Spanish "rain") seem to reflect the ideal of weightlessness. Lightness can be contrasted with at least one nickname from the collection of nature nicknames, although it neither fits neatly into the flora, fauna, nor the meteorology/astrology categories. *Sumpferl* (German "small swamp"), in terms of demeanor, is small but not light and rather depressing sounding. In this context, the metaphorical denotation of swamp suggests a person who is being sucked into the swamp and is perhaps beyond help. If "swamp" is seen as a metaphor for the eating disorder, this person does not

---

[51] One exception to avoiding connotations of bigness may be the nickname *Eta Carina*, which is the name of one of the largest known stars (see http://etacar.umn.edu/etainfo/). However, seen from the earth with the naked eye, any star is just a shiny dot in the sky, which at least puts its heaviness and bigness into perspective. Furthermore, the distinctive character of this nickname (it is very original) and the likelihood that HO participants do not know its original referent (i.e., the specific star) will not consider this potential exception very significant.

appear to have much hope in finding a cure. The nickname *Schatten-voegelchen* (German "small shadow bird") also does not seem very hopeful or positive, which, aside from its smallness and probably lightness, displays characteristics of hiding and possibly depression.

Personal nouns

A number of personal nouns are also used as nicknames. Almost all of them are female; only *Blue Guy*, which suggests a rather depressed persona because of the use of "blue," is male. Furthermore, it must be noted that many of the personal noun (phrase) nicknames tend to be self-depreciative. Consider the nickname *Ampelweibchen* (German "small traffic light female"). This is a modification of the term *Ampelmännchen* (German "small traffic light male"), which is a well-known (and nowadays even commercialized) figure that appears on German traffic lights. In fact, the little man *is* the traffic light, turning red and green. In terms of attributes, the characteristic of constantly changing colors suggests an unstable mind or a person that frequently changes her mind or does not know what she wants (which is slightly self-deprecating). With the nickname *Pueppi23* (German "small doll," which in this context can be read as "silly, over-dressed woman"), the actor is ascribed the derogatory features "silly" and "over-dressed." *Kellerkind* (German "cellar child") obviously denotes a child, and, when referring to a teenager, adolescent, or adult, projects the characteristics of a child onto the actor. *Kellerkind* as an actor-focal emblem invokes attributes such as scared, hiding, small, dark, and helpless. Adopting a nickname which is either an emblem for a silly, over-dressed woman, or a person who constantly changes her mind, together with references to oneself as a "child," implies a critical evaluation of the self or lack of self-esteem. The words *Pueppi* and *weibchen*, which explicitly denote women, are both derogatory.

In contrast to these nicknames, which display negative or self-deprecating personal attributes, stands a nickname like **+*SaLTaTriX_NiViS*+** (Latin "female snow dancer"). A stereotypical reading of this nickname yields personal identity attributes such as gracious, light, soft, pure, and distinctive. There is one personal noun that not only constructs a distinctive identity, but a potentially *self-confident* one: *quorkepf*. At first sight, this does not appear to be a personal noun, but when read as a modification of *Querkopf* (German "awkward customer"), it can be seen as an emblem of stubbornness or obstinacy (see next section).

"Eating disordered" nicknames

I have related the "small" and "light" nicknames to characteristics of eating disorders, but none of the nicknames in the corpus *literally* denotes food or eating behavior, most likely because nicknames that do so have been filtered out by the HO moderators. However, in the practice of "reading people," there are a few nicknames that can nevertheless be linked to eating disorder practices. *Schattenvoegelchen* (German "small shadow bird") evokes an image of the body of a particular participant. The "shadow" in this nickname implies secrecy, as if this individual can lurk and go unseen, but also a glimpse of a body, perhaps an emaciated body, an anorectic body, the result of starvation. In this manner and in this context, an eating disordered body can be read in this nickname. The second notable example is *Hamsterbacke* (German "greedy, voracious person," but literally "hamster cheek"). This is the only nickname that can be considered to directly embody a symptom of disturbed eating behavior, namely binging.

Loewen_maeulchen (German "snapdragon," but literally "small lion's mouth") similarly incorporates two layers of meaning that are both connected to the forum. On the one hand, a plant's name is not unusual in this forum and usually denotes nature, as, for instance, with *marienblume* (German "daisy"). On the other hand, the *maeulchen* (German "small mouth") has a tongue-in-cheek connotation with regard to eating disorders. A lion's mouth could be characterized as typical of an obese person, but the fact that it is a *small* lion's mouth may instead mean someone with a restrained eating behavior, as in anorexia. Certain personal attributes can also be linked to eating disorders and personality traits from the other nicknames (see section 5.6).

Famous referents

Almost half of the proper names in the corpus have famous or well-known referents (see table 4). This is noteworthy, since the Rules and Regulations state that nicknames cannot be identical to the name of another person, institution, or registered brand. Taken literally, any commonly known name would be forbidden based on this rule, but it appears that the rule is not always followed. It seems that participants sometimes succeed in getting their nicknames with certain types of well-known referents approved. However, the names of actresses, super models, pop singers, etc. are largely absent, probably because they are often rejected based on this rule. (*Brooke*, with its referent a figure from the soap opera *The Bold and the Beautiful* and/or the actress *Brooke Shields*, is an exception, probably because it has more than one famous referent.) Certain names of non-living or "unreal" referents appear to be tolerated. These include names of historical or mythical figures (e.g., *hypathia*, *Kassiopaiah*, *Anthea*, *Nikolaus*), well known personae from literary works, visual art, theater, or music (for example *Rusalka*, a famous opera by *Antonin Dvorak*, *Mona Lisa*, and *Salome*), and names of contemporary cartoon figures or film characters (e.g., *Schuenga* – a character from the German version of the movie *Nell*, *schnoopy* – similar to Snoopy, the famous dog from the Peanuts comic strip and cartoons, and *Dorie* – a cartoon character from the movie *Finding Nemo*). Each of these names, when read as an emblem, projects specific attributes of the referent of the name onto the participant who registered the name. I will give two examples. The name *hypathia* refers to a Greek female mathematician and philosopher and may be read as an emblem of wisdom and intelligence. However, *Hypathia* is also the name of a feminist philosophy journal, which makes the name a feminist emblem. Second, *Schuenga* is the pet form of the word *Schutzengel* (German "guardian angel") and invokes not only a guardian angel, but also the wish to have a guardian angel. In general, names of Greek goddesses or historical individuals are frequent. Attributes stereotypically associated with these Greek and other mythological or historical figures are noble, dignified, gracious, beautiful, and intelligent.

Contemporary	Historical
Dorie (cartoon figure)	Salome (daughter of Herodias)
schnoopy (cf. Snoopy)	Aletheia (goddess of truth)
lillifee79 (toy figure)	Anthea (epithet of Hera)
Pinkpanther (cartoon figure)	hypathia (mathematician and philosopher)

Table 4. Examples of famous referent nicknames

How could these historical figures be linked to eating disorders? Eating disorders are not just a disorder of puberty, an attempt to remain a girl, or the denial of one's femininity. Orbach claimed that the anorectic woman is not just weak and childish, but also "a crafty, strong and unyielding opponent" (2001: 4) in the struggle for power over who controls an individual woman's body. This strength can be read in distinctive, dignified nicknames such as *Kassiopaiah*, *Freya*, and *Aletheia*. These noble female Greek figures do not subscribe to the image of a child-like, small, or weightless being. However, the famous referents, mostly goddesses, artistic personae, or women of great stature, can also be seen as examples of the high expectations sufferers have of themselves or the goals they set for themselves: To become people of status who have achieved great things. In other words, these nicknames seem to symbolize aspirations rather than describe current realities.

As with "nature" nicknames, smallness as an attribute extends across the domains of both denotation and famous referents. Famous names with "small" referents include the cartoon figures, but also *lillifee79*, which refers to *Lillifee*, a small toy figure who takes care of animals. One commonly known proper name even has a diminutive ending, namely *Windjulchen*, composed of the German for "wind" and the name *Julie* with the diminutive *-chen*. Hence, many HO participants use their nicknames to present themselves as "small" people.

5.6 Analysis person attributes: Feminine, childish, depressed, distinctive or self-confident

Grouping the nicknames' personal attributes reveals that some seem to occur more frequently in the corpus: Femininity, childishness, depression, distinctiveness, and self-confidence. Femininity, as in femaleness, can be constructed through gender-coded emblems such as in *Ms.Dust*, since *Ms.* is coded as referring to a female. Additionally, however, certain stereotypical social images of femininity can be discerned in nicknames. With regard to personal attribute displayed through stereotypes, it appears that femininity is displayed in at least three variants: Nature femininity, childish femininity, and noble femininity. The connection of nature and femininity was already considered in the previous section. The Greek female referents are rather gracious, noble women, whereas the contemporary female cartoon/toy figures construct a childish kind of femininity, which is characterized by sweetness and cuteness. The absence of prototypical emblems of the sort of femininity related to beauty or attractiveness should not be mistaken for disinterest on the part of HO participants; these nicknames were probably rejected by the forum moderators because of the rule that prohibits nicknames of an offensive, confusing, insinuating, or acrimonious nature. Only two nicknames seem to display stereotypically feminine features or commodities related to beauty or attractiveness: *lillifee79* and *la careta* (Spanish "make up").

Another observation is that among the HO members there are no "sexually colored" nicknames at all, which is notable since in a forum for teenagers in the US, many "sexual" nicknames were found by Subrahmanyam et al. (2004). Even though at least a portion of the HO population belongs to that same age group, HO members do not use nicknames such as *Sugarbabe* or *Sexyqueen*. This could be explained by the members' avoidance of sexuality, which is considered a fairly common feature among eating-disordered women (Treasure et al., 2005). Alternatively, the HO moderators consider sexually colored nicknames offensive or acrimonious (because sexuality is presumably problematic for many members) and therefore reject such nicknames.

The attribute childish, in the HO context, evokes a certain type of femininity, with an emphasis on immaturity. Nicknames such as *Kitekati* (cf. English "kitty cat"), *Daisymaus* (English/German "daisy mouse") and *baerli* (German "small bear") are childish and accordingly, as argued above, stereotypically feminine. Women have frequently been characterized as childish (cf. Friedan, 1966/1963). Women are also more likely to be addressed as girls than men are to be addressed boys (Eckert and McConnell-Ginet, 2003). For this reason, in the current analysis, the attributes childish and feminine are assumed to overlap to a considerable extent.

A possible explanation for "childish" nicknames is that being like a child is related to the wish not to grow up. Growing up to be an adult woman is a painful experience for many eating disordered teenage girls. A girl's first menstruation experience can be fairly negative. It may be experienced as a loss of control, or worse, the body going "out of control." Orbach (2001: 132) recounts a case of an 11-year old that was told that her menstruation had started so early because she was a "big girl." The girl reacted by resolving that she would become a smaller girl by following a strict diet, which then made her period disappear for a number of years. This attempt to control the body can be described as "desexualizing" the female body. By reducing one's hips and breasts, and eliminating her period, a girl can ignore or reduce essential aspects of adult femininity.

The attribute depressed or being down can be read from a number of the nicknames, both among the nature nicknames and others. *Blue Guy* and *Masnie*, which has no denotation, but reads backwards as *einsam* (German "lonely"), ascribe the attribute "depressed" to its referent. The persona attribute of being down or depressed may be linked to the co-morbidity of eating disorders and depression (Fornari et al., 1992). Orbach relates depression to self-hate, the term she prefers to describe eating disordered people's low self-esteem. "Self hate is debilitating. Anyone who suffers it will do almost anything to disguise it. They [*sic*] may turn into depression" (Orbach, 2001: 112). This means that self-deprecating nicknames have similar traits as those alluding to depression. It must be stressed, however, that nicknames that convey the attribute depression are very few in this sample, possibly because these have been rejected by the HO moderators or because depressed people were less likely to respond to the study's call for respondents.

The attribute distinctiveness expresses the characteristic of being special or exceptional in a positive sense. Creativity is, to a certain extent, always required when choosing or constructing a nickname. This is because many nicknames have already been registered (each nickname can only be used once), or because, according to the HO rules, the nicknames cannot be identical to the name of another person, institution, or registered brand. With the attribute distinctiveness, however, I mean more than creativity, since it is also related to exclusiveness, refinement, and dignity. For example, in HO, a Spanish nickname like *tortuga* (Spanish "turtle") is more distinctive than the German equivalent. Thus, distinctive in the present analysis is meant as original, for instance, in choice of language. Novel formations can also be read as distinctive, as can names of certain famous referents. The great variety of languages and the effect of a non-German nickname as being different, distinctive, or even dignified may be linked to the desire to be unlike everyone else, a dream of being someone special, which is something that is evident in many sufferers (Bruch, 2001). The multilingualism in nicknames may also be a sign of globalization, not in the sense of the English-speaking "global village" or one dominant world culture (Bechar-Israeli, 1995), but as a reflection of the participants' awareness of, and openness toward, other languages and cultures. Alternatively, the fact that the interaction in the forum is exclusively in German suggests that using a foreign language to create one's nickname is a way to make one's online identity special or exotic.

Self-confidence can be read as a personal attribute in only a few nicknames. The nickname *quorkepf* was mentioned previously, but also *krats*, which, when read backwards is *stark* (German "strong"), seems to evoke self-confidence or strength. Furthermore, **Vivo** (Italian "I live") can be considered positive when read as: "I am happy to be alive" or "I am happy to be living!" However, all of these cases could also be read as emblematic of the opposite. **Vivo** can also be read as: "I am barely alive anymore." Additionally, since "stark" and "Querkopf" have been modified (i.e., the e and o have been swapped in *quorkepf*, and the word is completely reversed in *krats*), the self-confidence is debatable because it has been modified or obscured. The self-confident nicknames *quorkepf* and *krats* do not reflect childishness, either. However, the modifications, as discussed above, are noteworthy. A possible explanation is that participants see the HO forum as a social community where a manifestation of strength is inappropriate. It has been noted that girls suffering from anorexia "struggle with the challenge to claim their strengths without 'sounding like a bitch/a snob/stuck up'" (Bruch, 2000: xvi). However, whether this is the explanation for the modifications in these names remains speculative.

The recurring personal attributes that nicknames as emblems convey can be visualized as circles that overlap (figure 2). One nickname can be a sign of various attributes, depending on how the nickname is read. *Kellerkind* has been argued to construct both a depressed and childish attribute, *Schatten-voegelchen* both depressed and feminine, etc.

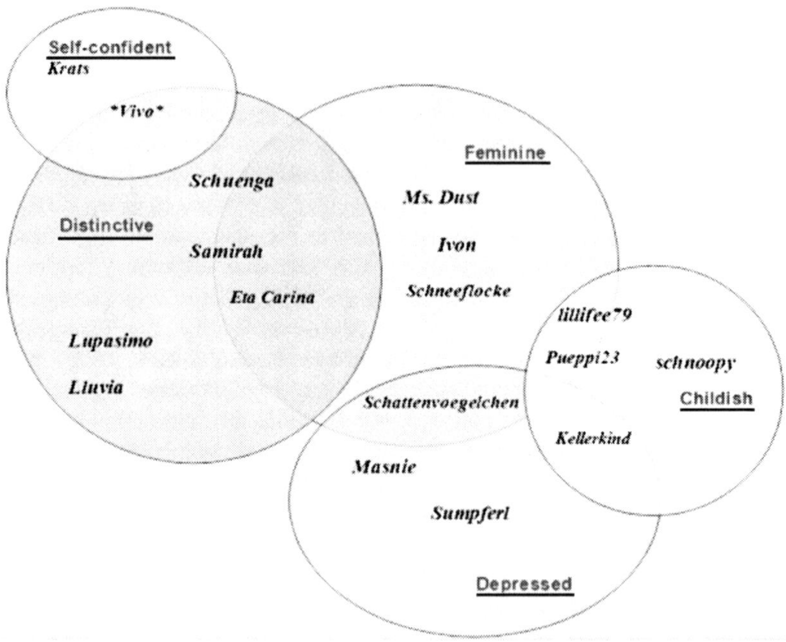

Fig.2. Personal attributes in nicknames

5.7 Conclusion

For a proper understanding of the relevancies of entering an online support group, nicknames have been considered, especially as entities that construct identity. In an anonymous forum, it is mainly nicknames that establish the participants' identity and, therefore, these nicknames create certain impressions or apparent faces of the various HO members. The analysis of nicknames therefore shows certain traits or attributes HO members articulate for their presence on the forum.

The analysis demonstrated various directions in which nicknames (read as emblems) characterize their referents. Some recurring personal attributes are smallness, weightlessness (snow, wind, star, etc.), childishness (e.g., cartoon figures), and depression or negative self-evaluation, but also noble femininity (names of Greek goddesses and historical individuals). Many of these attributes are traditionally associated with femininity, which reveals how nicknames can be gendered in a non-apparent, largely metaphorical manner. Many of the attributes in nicknames have been argued to be plausibly related to eating disorders.

Mapping the nicknames and personal attributes of eating disordered people is not intended to essentialize aspects of the self or personhood of the individuals suffering from a severe illness; rather, it is an attempt to understand the role nicknames play in online identity construction. It appears that nicknames should not only be considered as medium-specific linguistic forms, but also as signs that derive signification from their contexts. This means that it would be inaccurate to advance typologies of nicknames without considering the online setting.

Furthermore, the analysis raises questions about forum policy regarding the constitution of nicknames. It has been demonstrated that, despite forum rules, participants register nicknames that can be read as conveying various attributes of personhood, and which thus construct online personae. HO participants express the personal relevance or importance of their nickname in forum interactions. One participant emphasized that if she got better at some point, she would need a new nickname. Since the forum's aim is to overcome eating disorders, it can be argued that sufferers, in the process of recovery, should have the option to change their nicknames. For example, when *Sumpferl* (German "small swamp") ultimately begins to head on her way toward recovery and feels more optimistic, she will probably want a more positive nickname. A list of previous nicknames for each participant would avoid problems in recognizing HO participants. Therefore, the possibility of nickname change should be (re)considered by the HO association.

Chapter 6

Opening the first posting: Ambivalence towards the community

6.1 Introduction

The opening lines of first postings are the focus of attention in this chapter. The virtual entrance to the forum by novice members is frequently articulated by the construction of the novice member as insecure or uncertain. This means that the novice member typically begins her/his first posting by displaying her/himself as hesitant or lacking in confidence. Other forum members respond almost ritualistically by offering a "warm" welcome and reassuring the novice member by emphasizing her/his courage in daring to join the forum in the first place. Reassurance is sometimes accompanied by statements about the nature of the forum. First, I will demonstrate that insecurity is enacted both through content (i.e., verbalization) and features of oral discourse, which enables the novice to convey ambivalent or slightly contradictory stances about joining the HO forum. This means that becoming a member of HO is discursively articulated as a difficult step. Second, I will show that insecure openings seem to encourage welcomes, but also reassurance and appreciation from regular members. The third part of the analysis focuses on the issues of identity and community in opening postings. It scrutinizes the facets of identities enacted here and reveals that a discursive construction of the community can again signal the novices' ambivalence about becoming a member but can also be employed by regulars not only to reassure or appreciate novices, but even to resolutely include them if their ambivalence seems to be based on "false" grounds, such as someone's denial of actually having an eating disorder.

Openings are not considered merely structural features of postings, but as crucial environments in forum interactions for the enactment of identities and community features. Openings in online interactions have received very little research attention thus far, and most of it has been focused on chat openings rather than forum interactions (e.g., Rintal et al., 2001). Since there *are* various CA studies that investigate phone call openings, I will explore these to come to a distinction of various types of identity that play a role in phone calls. The review of the studies that investigate phone calls leads to an idea of what identity in openings of forum conversation may encompass. Since first postings generally receive a response that involves various aspects of the first posting, responses are included in the analysis. Moreover, there is a methodological reason to include responses. Applying the *next turn proof procedure* (Hutchby and Wooffitt, 1991), responses may ratify the reading of the first posting. First, however, I will explore how openings can be demarcated from "the body" of postings as consisting of subject lines, greetings and prefaces. Before I present the analysis of HO openings, I will explain the types of identities that are relevant in phone call openings.

6.2 Defining openings and exploring the relevance of identity

This chapter examines openings of first postings and the response by a second participant in relation to the opening. Therefore, a definition of what a CMC forum opening consists of structurally and an elaboration on why the first reply is an important point to analyze in this regard are needed.

Subject lines

Subject lines or thread titles are produced by the person who initiates the thread, and are placed at the top of the posting, followed by the nickname of the author. Subject lines can be seen as setting the tone or theme so that the reader will understand the subsequent text in a certain way. However, subject lines do not only appear in the thread itself but also in the *overview* of threads in the forum (see figure 3).

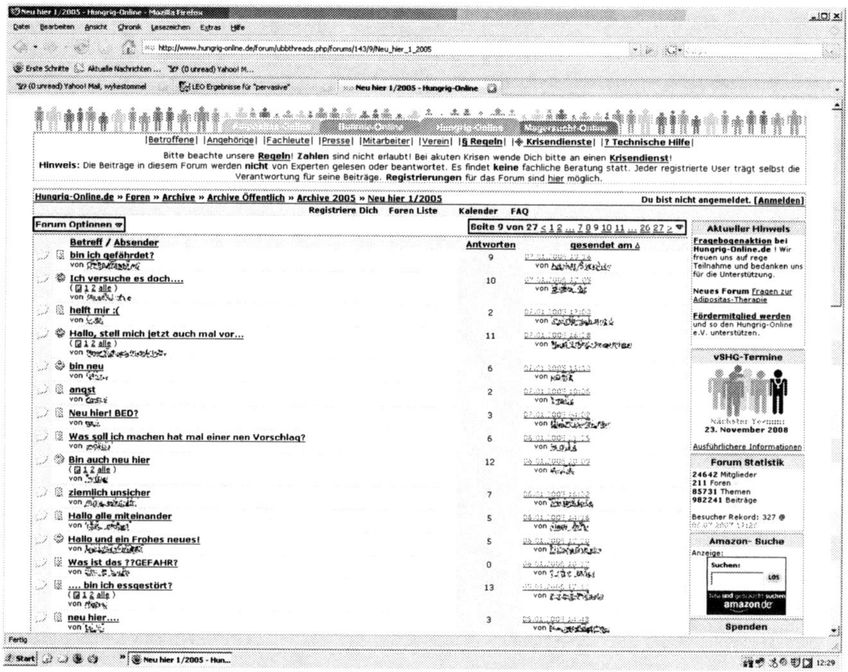

Fig. 3. Overview of subject lines from the HO forum (nicknames are made illegible)

Readers actually gain access to the thread by clicking on the subject line, which makes the thread appear on the screen. Thus, they are not only the opening of a posting, but they are the labels of the whole thread, and the first visible indication of theme offered to potential readers. In other words, subject lines are crucial for those reading the thread (Antaki et al., 2005; Stegbauer, 2000), since the title's appeal determines which users will open the thread. The HO Rules and Regulations recommend using a significant formulation for the subject line, so instead of "I have a question..." they recommend "Question about cognitive therapy," which actually announces a theme. This shows that subject lines are considered fairly important by the HO management, but it remains unclear to what extent members take this rule into account while formulating a subject line.

Greetings

Graphically, the first posting of the thread commences to the right of the subject line and the authors' nickname. Most first postings start with a greeting, varying in (in)formality from *Hallo* to *Hallo Ihr Lieben*. Previous research showed that greetings can play a role in community solidarity and community construction in CMC (Thimm and Ehmer, 2000). Research on workplace email exchanges has shown that greetings (or salutations) and closings serve an important function in the constructing and maintaining of relationships (e.g., Waldvogel, 2007). They can express warmth or distance but they can also reinforce status relationships (position in the professional hierarchy) and underline positional expectations. Waldvogel (2007) found that greetings and closings were used to construct solidarity more often in messages sent to groups than to individual colleagues. She concluded that the absence or presence of greetings and closings in an organization's emails provides insights into its culture. In fact, the workplace culture was discovered to depend more on greetings and closings than on the sociolinguistic variables of status, social distance, and gender of the interlocutors. These findings suggest that openings and closings in asynchronous forum conversation may also play a role in terms of social relations. The present study, however, does not include an analysis of the socio-cultural data of the participants (for ethical reasons, see section 4.3). Hence, it focuses solely on the discursive practices, excluding sociolinguistic variables and ethnographic studies including interviews regarding culture. Thus, openings and closings are considered structural features that may be consequential for the course of the interaction and simultaneously co-constitutive of identities and the community.

Prefaces of first postings and the next turn

A first reading of the various HO threads in the New Here forum revealed that participants often produce "something else" before introducing themselves. The "something else" that precedes the actual off-take of a story is called a *preface* (Sacks, 1974). A preface operates as a key to understanding the subsequent text in a certain way (Antaki et al., 2005). Sacks has noted that prefaces are powerful tools, because they send a signal to the next speaker about the classification of eventual reactions that would be consistent with the material in the upcoming story, such as appreciation or sympathy (Sacks, 1992: vol. 1 p. 682; vol. 2, p.10, cit. in Antaki et al., 2005).

I will elaborate in a little more detail what Antaki et al. (2005) concluded about the use of a preface in a forum discussion in order to show that the next turn (i.e., the response) can or should be read as a ratification of the first turn, despite the fact that turn organization in CMC is notably different from that found in spoken interaction. In their data, a member of the involved forum announces a "declaration of love" as a preface. The posting is composed by someone calling herself Lourdes and opens like this:

> Lourdes:
>
> Para ella, que ya sabe quién es, con todo mi amor
> ('For she, who already knows who she is, with all my love').
>
> Source: Antaki et al. (2005: n.p.).

What follows is a poem, conventionally known as a love poem. The header or subject line of the posting is *Para ella, que sabe quién es* ("For she, who knows who she is") which is repeated, but further specified as *ya* ("already") in the first line of the posting (see above). Leaving aside the analysis of this announcement in the subject line, the focus will be on the subsequent *con todo mi amor* ("with all my love"). The authors understood it as a preface, and thus as setting the tone for a response that will be consistent with the positive emotion implied by someone who offers something with all one's love.[52] The first response to Lourdes' posting is consistent with the preface of the first posting, which implies that the recipient (named London_derry) has indeed read *con todo mi amor* as a preface. She typed:

> London_derry:
>
> Vaya manera de poneros los dientes largos, chiquilla... Poz ná, a aguantarse, digo!!!! Muakis a las dos
>
> ('What a way to make us green with envy, girlie... well, we're gonna have to live with it, I guess!!! Kissy-kiss to both of you').
>
> Source: Antaki et al. (2005: n.p.).

According to Antaki et al., in terms of adjacency pairs, this response (i.e., the next turn) treats Lourdes's posting as a first part that calls up *appreciation* as an appropriate second part. In other words, Lourdes's posting is not treated as inappropriate (because it is a personal message not meant for the whole community), but as something to be appreciated. This shows that the analysis of the replies to first postings is helpful for understanding what happened in the first posting, since they reveal how the first posting was treated by others.

To summarize, the present analysis defines openings as encompassing subject lines, greetings and prefaces that appear prior to the "body" of the posting. In some cases, also the ending of the posting is considered. The relationship between openings and responses is relevant, since the next turn may display a reading of the first turns' opening.

Openings and identity in calls

There is reason to expect that identity will be especially relevant in the openings of the HO threads, especially when we compare them to phone conversations. Typically in phone conversations, after the summon-answer se-

[52] The end of Lourdes' posting is a restatement of the opening material, signaling that what the preface promised has been delivered. According to Antaki et al. (2005), this is common for turns which have begun with a preface. In other words, postings with a preface may have an ending with a restatement of what was written in the opening.

quence, an identification or recognition of the caller and recipient follows. Schegloff stated:

> Whatever a telephone conversation is going to be occupied with, however bureaucratic or intimate, routine or unusual, earthshaking or trivial, it and its parties will have to pass through the identification/recognition sieve as the first thing they do (1979: 71).

Consider the following excerpt of a canonical opening of a call:

Prior:	Hello?
Irene:	Doctor Prior?
Prior:	Yes,
Irene:	Irene Davis.
Prior:	Yes Irene.
Irene:	Good morning. =

Source: Schegloff (1986: 137).

This example displays various types of identity. Most obviously, the identities of the individuals are accomplished by announcing one's name, which is the case at least in formal phone calls. Second, Irene addresses the respondent by adding the title to his name ("Doctor Prior"), and thereby performs an identity category (doctor), implicitly making relevant what is socially known about the category "doctor." It is important to note that the identities displayed by names are simultaneously indications or constituents of the relationship. As Schegloff put it:

> [O]ne issue potentially addressed in conversation openings is the reconstitution of the parties' relationship – who they are to one another, the current state of the relationship, and the relationship between the current, incipient occasion of interaction and prior one(s) (1968: 140).

In this sense, the identities that are performed are always situation-bound. However, conversation analysts have often chosen to understand situation as message-intrinsic (Hopper, 1992: 72). From an ethnomethodological point of view, they are interested in local practices, or how participants display situational relevancies to one another. Participants may focus on the message-extrinsic aspects, such as gender, intimacy and culture, but is it neither presumed that these factors are per definition relevant to the conversation, nor that they determine the interaction. Hopper (1992: 80) has provided the example of a woman calling a pizza delivery service and opening with: "Hi honey, how ya doin hih?," which is in direct contrast to the "canonical" fashion of institutional or formal calls, or calls between strangers. Therefore, the situation must be understood as produced during the conduct of conversation. Zimmerman stressed that

> the opening of the call, and in particular, the first component or components of the first turn of the answerer and caller are regularly devoted to establishing a mutually oriented-to set of identities implicative for the shape of what is to follow (1998: 98).

Hence, the situation of a conversation cannot be defined a priori. But still, calls between strangers routinely follow a certain format and different types of calls seem to have their own unique formats. Consider radio phone-ins, where the situation is such that the caller already knows the identity of the respondent (the radio show host). A summon-answer sequence is not produced (at least not "on air"), and the identification-recognition sequence is not achieved in the routine form of a sequence. Generally, it is argued that in radio phone-in conversations, the *situational* identity of host and caller are consequential to the course of interaction (Fitzgerald and Housley, 2002; Hutchby, 2000). In other words, the host and caller opposition is grounded in the institutional setting and the division of labor defining the two situational roles. These identities are usually established during the opening sequences of the interaction.

Although CMC interactions differ from telephone conversations in substantial ways (e.g., in text-only CMC voice recognition is impossible, the organization of turns is different), it can be assumed that participants' identities in relation to the situation are also relevant here. The role of greetings in CMC has already been mentioned as constitutive of relationships, but situational identities, such as novice and regular member can also be relevant in forum openings, similar to the doctor-identity in the phone call above. Moreover, as first postings are usually more directed at a group of readers (the forum community) than at any one particular reader, not only are the individuals' identities "oriented to" or accomplished but the community as a whole as well.

6.3 Goal

The general objective is to map the relevant aspects of the openings of first postings. The aim is to analyze the characteristics of those openings in terms of identities and community. Important questions are: Do members create relevant identities and community in openings? How do novice members orient to situational identities (such as novice or regular)? How do they address the forum? How do regulars treat the novice? How do regulars respond to those openings?

The analysis of openings is presented in three sections. Section 6.4 focuses on the characteristics of insecurity/hesitancy in openings. It examines how insecurity is enacted in openings, both through verbalization and through the employment of typical oral features. Subsequently, section 6.5 investigates how recipients' replies can be seen as a response to the insecure openings, seemingly in terms of an adjacency pair. Regulars tend to welcome and reassure the insecure novice member. Section 6.6 shows how identities and the community are enacted and employed to do certain things in openings.

Note that:

- Nicknames are replaced by pseudonyms, and age is replaced by age groups for the sake of anonymity.
- Text inside brackets in the excerpts is either anonymized information added by the author (W.S.) or the description of an emoticon/smiley.
- The excerpt codes (#...) refer to the unique position of data in the data set.
- The typing, spelling and punctuation are taken from the originals.
- The English translations of postings are added for the sake of comprehension, but the original German messages are the actual research material.

6.4 Analysis: Insecurity in openings of first postings

First postings that open a new thread in the New Here sub-forum reveal that members often "do" some kind of insecurity, hesitancy or doubt, which sometimes also encompasses a reference to the registration and having read other members' postings before actually composing one. This phenomenon of lurking before joining a forum has been frequently observed (Preece et al., 2004). Consider, for instance, the following opening by Irene (^_^ = "smiley face").

Irene:
Hey, I'm new and stuff^_^;
… And I suck at making topics like this
I've been lurking here a while now, and decided to finally
register …

Source: Benwell and Stokoe (2006: 268).

Upon first observation, we see that Irene is explicitly constructing herself as a "newbie," which is an identity relevant to the situation, and which is, as in phone calls, performed at the very beginning of the contribution. The sentence *I've been lurking here a while now, and decided to finally register* is a reference to the common activity of lurking before joining. Benwell and Stokoe considered this sentence as typical of the "widely observed phenomenon that newbies 'do' being cautious" (2006: 273). This comment stresses that this novice member has not registered spontaneously, but only after having lurked for some time. Thus, it constructs the novice member as equitable and reasonable, which is someone who has prepared her/his initiation into the community.[53] In this section, I will demonstrate that this type of cautiousness in openings of HO postings is enacted in a more extreme fashion, namely not only by being cautious, but even insecure, hesitant or unsure. I will eventually analyze what "doing insecurity" is used for, or helps to achieve.

Various methods of doing insecurity can be distinguished. In the first place, insecurity is performed by directly verbalizing it, either naming the insecurity, naming the courage that is required to write a posting or expressing ignorance or uncertainty regarding the content or location of the posting. In the second place, insecurity can be done through a display of the ongoing production of language by means of features of oral discourse, such as pauses (ellipses) and other cues such as *Hm* and *Naja* (Well) but also a reflective style. These features evoke doubt or uncertainty with regard to the contradictory, sometimes paradoxical, statements, feelings and opinions expressed by the novice member.

The following section focuses solely on openings (subject lines, greetings, prefaces and some endings of first postings) and distinguishes between verbalizing insecurity and expressing it through oral discourse features.

---

[53] With Sacks (1992), it could be claimed that "doing" being cautious at the beginning of one's participation in an online group is an instance of "doing" being ordinary. "Doing" being ordinary refers to the job that people have in their world, "as their constant preoccupation" (Sacks, 1992: 216), to do being ordinary. The question following from this assumption is how people do this, how they go about having usual interests, usual thoughts, etc. For joining a forum, it seems to be the ordinary way to start your posting by mentioning that you have lurked a while and then decided to register (thus countering that you joined spontaneously, without having looked around first), by which you achieve being an ordinary person.

Verbalizing insecurity

The verbalized insecurity can be related to what the member feels s/he should write, or whether s/he is in the right place (appropriate forum) for her/his concern. Consider excerpts 1-4. Note that the subject lines of excerpt 3 and 4 directly display this insecurity.

Excerpt 1 (#33)

Antonia: Hallo bin neu…
Hallo ihr,
Ich bin noch ein bisschen unsicher was ich schreiben soll. [...]

Antonia: Hello, I'm new...
Hello you guys,
I'm still a bit unsure about what I should write. [...]

Excerpt 2 (#31)

Sylvia: bin ich gefährdet?
hallo ihr forumaner…
also eigentlich weiss ich gar nicht genau was ich hier schreiben soll […]

Sylvia: am I at risk?
hello you forumers...
so, i don't actually know what i should write here exactly [...]

Excerpt 3 (#22)

Doreen: ziemlich unsicher
Hallo mal an all!
Ich bin mir nicht wirklich sicher ob ich hier richtig bin, […]

Doreen: quite unsure
Hi everyone!
I'm not really sure if I'm in the right place, [...]

Excerpt 4 (#7)

Katrina: bin ich hier wohl richtig?
Hallo erstmal.

also ich habe mir ziemlich lange überlegt, ob ich mich hier anmelden soll oder nicht.
[…]

Katrina: am I in the right place?
First of all: hello.
so I contemplated for quite a long time about whether I should register here or not.
[…]

Not knowing what to write or not knowing whether you are in the right place are ways of expressing apprehension or insecurity about being in a particular forum. It suggests that certain things should not be written, or that certain individuals may not be in the right place – in HO – and/or that the member her/himself is actually shy, careful, or uncertain. In other words, novice members, in the opening of their postings, do not treat HO as a low-threshold online space where any concern with regard to eating disorders is equally appreciated or taken seriously. In some cases, it is not the insecurity itself that is formulated, but the *courage* which is required to post for the first time. Consider excerpts 5-6.

Excerpt 5 (#2)
Veronika: N'abend…
So, nun trau ich mich auch mal  […]

Veronika: Evening…
So, now I'll also be brave  *[…]*

Excerpt 6 (#17)
Martine: neu hier…
Hallo,
angemeldet bin ich schon eine ganze Weile, aber erst habe ich nicht den Mut gefunden zu schreiben und dann ist die registrierung wieder in Vergessenheit geraten.
Nun aber endlich…
Kurz zu mir: […]

Martine: new here…
Hello,
I've already been signed up for quite a while, but I couldn't find the courage to write at first and then the registration was forgotten.

But now, finally...
About me: [...]

By explaining that writing requires courage, these members point out that the writing of a first posting in HO is a big step for them. They sometimes refer to the time it has taken them to actually post a contribution (excerpts 4, 5 and 6), which either displays the time needed to summon the courage (excerpts 5 and 6), in relation to shame (the emoticon in excerpt 5) or they have expressed doubt about joining the forum (excerpt 4). In sum, by verbalizing insecurity, novice members construct themselves as hesitant or as lacking confidence, but they also imply that is not that easy to become a member of HO.

Doing insecurity through features of oral discourse

The second way to display insecurity is through the employment of oral discourse features. That CMC is in some respects more like spoken conversation, than like written discourse has already been argued by Yates (1996), for instance. Rather than defining CMC as a medium distinct from spoken and written language, I will here focus on the interactional actions that are usually conducted through the use of oral features in CMC. For this purpose, *typical* oral and *typical* written discourse features must be distinguished (Jahandarie, 1999), which leaves room for genre-specific (or individual) cases, in which the dichotomy is overlooked, such as personal notes (more features of oral than written discourse) or academic lectures (sometimes displaying more written than oral features).

For the analysis, the relevant typical features are presented in table 5.

	Speaking	Writing
1	Prosodic	Punctuated
2	Evanescent	Permanent
3	Contextualized	Autonomous
4	Involved	Detached
5	Redundancy	Concise
6	Transparent	Dense
7	Fuzzy	Precise

Table 5. Features of oral vs. written discourse, Jahandarie (1999: 131-150).

I will explain these features briefly. Prosody refers to intonation and emphasis, whereas punctuation refers to capitalization, italicization and bold facing (producing emphasis) as well as question marks, exclamation points, ellipsis and periods (performing intonation). Generally, prosody and punctuation are similar means to the same end, but prosody generally appears to be more effective than punctuation. The second feature indicates the ephemeral character of speech in contrast to the permanence of writing. Thirdly, speech is more contextualized with respect to the physical situation in terms of deixis than written discourse, while the written text is more autonomous in the sense that it can be understood more independently of the situation. As a consequence, authors tend to contextualize within a text. A striking example of this is the fact that adolescent girls add contextualization to their diaries (unnecessarily so because the intended reader is only the writer herself), such as the precise locations of things, which are explained by the fact that writing typically invites contextual detail (Shuman, 1986). Fourth, speech displays more involvement than written text. Involvement consists of three components. Oral discourse displays greater:

- Involvement with the listener (the social activity of speaking, which may invoke intimacy and stance, or the speaker's positioning).
- Involvement with the self (personal pronouns, active voice, expressions of feelings and opinions and more extensive use of emphatic particles).
- Involvement with the here-and-now reality.

Accordingly, "in writing, the primary purpose is to convey information, not to establish a relationship" (Jahandarie, 1999: 139), which implies that conveying information is uninvolved.

The fifth feature covers the notion that in oral discourse we find more repetition and redundancy, while written discourse is more concise. Furthermore, speech is more transparent and less dense than written discourse:

> [It] moves ahead at about the same pace as the speaker's thoughts, thus capturing the on-going, almost *unedited thinking processes* much better than writing can. (Jahandarie, 1999: 145, emphasis added, W.S.).

In other words, spoken language shows a lot more about the process of its production than written language does. The last characteristic covers the notion that speech is fuzzier or less precise than written text, which may have to do with the fact that more time is spent in writing a message than actually speaking it. In speech, we use more fuzzy terms such as "like," "stuff" and "sort of" and non-explicit pronouns. The precision of writers is observed even when they write a first draft that no one will ever read. Overall, Biber has underscored that "it is possible, within each mode, to override the salient situational characteristics of the mode" (1988: 161), which is true, for instance, for personal letters. Having some oral characteristics, they aim to mimic a conversational style.

In the HO forum, the employment of oral features can be observed widely. The threads are frequently characterized by extreme uses of punctuation, little contextualization, and high levels of involvement, redundancy, transparency and fuzziness. Here, I would like to focus on the cases in which these oral features contribute to the enactment of insecurity. Very significantly, the ellipsis (...) is used extensively. It is a fairly unusual form of punctuation in typical written discourse and often suggests a "spoken" pause or it means that the rest of a thought will be understood and does not need to be stated. Members express insecurity or doubt via ellipses, as early as in the heading position of the posting: The subject line (see excerpts 1, 2, 5 and 6 above). The novice members implicitly mark the complete thread by employing this feature. The use of an ellipsis is also related to the oral feature of transparency. It articulates a pause in terms of time, and thus a display of the ongoing production (including silences) of the text.

The oral feature of transparency can refer to the "unedited thinking process," which can be displayed by a "thinking out loud" style. This is frequently used in first postings. Moreover, involvement is enacted in various ways, which is clearly observable in the next two excerpts. First consider excerpt 7.

Excerpt 7 (#18)
Debby: ... bin ich essgestört?
Hallo zusammen!
Vor einigen Tagen habe ich mich bei Euch im Forum angemeldet und nun sitze ich
hier vorm PC und überlege, ob ich mich trauen soll, Euch als Aussenstehende die
Frage zu stellen, ob ich eine Essstörung habe... wenn ich am Schluss den Beitrag ab-
schicke, dann hab ich mich getraut... wir werden sehen.
[...]
Jetzt habe ich so viel getippt und wird's nun auch abschicken. Ich hoffe, ich langweile
niemanden damit. [...]

Debby: ... do I have an eating disorder?
Hello everybody!
A few days ago, I signed up with you in the forum and now I'm sitting here in front of the computer, thinking about whether I dare to ask you as outsiders whether I have an eating disorder... if I send off this post at the end, then I'll have dared... we'll see.
[...]
Now I've typed so much and will actually send it off now. I hope I won't bore anybody with it. [...]

The formulation *ich überlege* (I am thinking, line 2-3) refers to a reflective act, which exhibits transparency rather than the (written) dense result of a thinking process. Thus, Debby employs an oral feature to present herself as thinking out loud. Furthermore, she uses ellipses within sentences, which can be interpreted both as pauses (related to the oral feature of prosody) and as instances that represent the thinking process (transparency). The sentence *wir werden sehen* (line 5) is a case of involvement, either with herself (in this case, "we'll see" is an idiom) or with the readers, when both Debby and the readers are included in the "we." Moreover, *wir werden sehen* refers to a here-and-now situation.

The ending to Debby's posting is also an enactment of the oral feature of involvement. *wird's nun auch abschicken* (line 7) shows involvement with the here and now (*nun* only makes sense in the here-and-now situation of typing the contribution), and the concern whether she bores the others shows her involvement with her readers. The assessment *Jetzt habe ich soviel getippt* displays involvement with the here and now, but is also a reference to potential redundancy.

All together, the oral features enable the writer to display characteristics of the on-going production of language. In this on-going process, the "I" can express contradictory thoughts, which is a form of doing insecurity. In excerpt 7, the contradiction follows. By writing what Debby was thinking of doing (i.e., posting), she, in fact, has already done what she is thinking of doing. Put differently, writing about considering to write something is a situation of the snake biting its own tail. The pauses expressed by ellipses add to that doubt and uncertainty. The display of doubt or insecurity about the question of whether she has an eating disorder may protect Debby from allegations about having asked it in the first place.

In excerpt 8, we again see how the oral features are put at work.

Excerpt 8 (#8)

Monique: Erste Annäherung

Hm, sehr merkwürdig, jetzt wirklich selbst etwas zu verfassen. Habe mich gestern schon registrieren lassen, wurde heute jedoch erst freigeschaltet und so hatte ich schon ein bisschen Zeit, mir die Beiträge von euch anderen durchzulesen. Manches erinnert mich sehr an mich, anderes ist mir völlig fremd. Aber bevor ich hier schreibe und schreibe: Hallo. Ich bin [18-22] Jahre

[…]

So, viel zu viel geschrieben, würde mich sehr froh, wenn mich jemand als Neuling hier begrüßen und mir schreiben würde!

Monique: First approach

Hm, very strange, now actually writing something myself. Got myself signed up yesterday, but was only activated today, and so I had a bit of time to read through the postings from you others. Some things reminded me a lot of myself, others are completely different. But before I write and write: Hello. I'm [18-22] years old

[…]

So, written much too much, would be very happy, since I'm a newcomer here, if somebody would say hello and write back to me!

Despite the fact that the subject line is typically written discourse (autonomous, detached, dense and precise), the *Hm* at the very beginning is a feature that constructs the posting as oral-like discourse. It is a sound that may be interpreted as doubt or thoughtfulness. In the first lines, Monique drops the personal pronoun "I" twice, which is a typical feature of oral discourse. The description of having lurked during the time between registration and having received one's login is not that concise, but rather self-involved and contextualized. Moreover, the duplication of *schreibe* (line 5) is redundant.

With regard to the oral/written dichotomy, it is notable that Monique types a colon, which marks the shift from the predominantly oral passage to a more autonomous and concise style, which resembles typical written discourse. Although a greeting displays involvement with others, this greeting is more concise than that of most other openings (such as *Hallo ihr*, *hallo ihr forumaner…*, *Hallo mal an alle!*, *Hallo erstmal*). The end of the posting is again quite oral (transparent and involved): *So, viel zu viel geschrieben* (line 8) as thinking out loud, a request for a response as other-involvement and *So* as reference to here-and-now.

Hence, as in excerpt 7, excerpt 8 displays the oral style that enables the poster to express doubt or contradiction in the sense of "on the one hand yes, on the other hand no." The sentence *Manches erinnert mich sehr an mich, anderes ist mir völlig fremd* (line 4-5) exhibits this most clearly. The insecurity, conveyed through oral features, is related to the fact that some things in HO seem familiar whereas other things are strange to Monique. The display of this yes/no position takes the form of oral discourse in terms of its ongoing, here-and-now process of production.

To conclude, the HO postings by novice members do insecurity through verbalizing it or more indirectly through employing oral features that enable the member to say one thing now and the opposite next. This insecurity makes it clear that posting a first contribution in HO is a big step and that both semantic and discourse-specific tools are employed to articulate this. The next section explores how other members respond to insecure novices.

6.5 Analysis: Insecurity – welcoming: An adjacency pair?

Messages are known to come in adjacency pairs. This is true for greetings, which stimulate reciprocal greetings, questions that require answers, invitations that require acceptances or refusals, etc. Generally, the characteristic of an adjacency pairs is that it consists of two utterances in sequential order, each produced by a different speaker. The pair is structured in a first part (e.g., question) and a second part (e.g., answer). What makes these pairs especially powerful devices is that the first part makes the second part *relevant* (Schegloff, 1968; Schegloff and Sacks, 1973). This means that when the first part occurs, the normative expectation is that the other speaker will produce the second part. If the second part is not produced, this is observable in what comes next in the conversation: Either the first speaker will repeat the first part louder, reformulate it, or eventually decide that the other person did not want to return the greeting, or respond to the question or summons (Houtkoop and Koole, 2000).

In asynchronous CMC, messages generally contain much more than just one conversational action (Herring, 1999). They contain greetings, questions, stories, good-byes, etc. all in one posting. This makes it hard to distinguish adjacency pairs, because adjacency can only be a criterion if the complete postings can be understood as one turn (e.g., Antaki et al., 2005). Antaki et al.

ratified their own reading of a first thread posting by reading the recipient posting as a second part of an adjacency pair, and thus as the relevant action in response to the first posting. In other words, they assume that a first posting and its response form an adjacency pair. They stated that the response "treats [the first] message as the kind of first part that calls up *appreciation* as an appropriate second part" (2005: n.p.), although they did not specify what kind of adjacency pair this is.

If a posting (one turn) contains a number of conversational actions, it is problematic to read the posting as one action (for instance appreciation). For example, in Ann's reply in excerpt 9, several actions are conducted.

Excerpt 9 (#16)

Ann (first response to Brenda)

Erstmal willkommen und schön, daß du dich hier meldest!
Wenn ich dich richtig verstehe fühlst du dich nicht "klassisch magersüchtig". Du reagierst nur mit Magenproblemen auf Streß aller Art und nimmst dadurch ab (so kurz zusammengefasst).
[…]
Nochmal: Ich finds toll, daß du etwas gegen deine Beschwerden tun willst!
Das beste ist echt eine Therapie. Mittelchen können nur Symptome lindern.
Liebe Grüße
Ann

Ann (first response to Brenda)
Firstly, welcome and it's great that you've signed up here!
If I understand you correctly, you don't feel "classically anorectic". You just react to stress with stomach problems of all kinds and therefore lose weight (to briefly sum it up).
[…]
Again: I think it's fantastic that you want to do something to help your condition!
The best thing really, is therapy. Medication can only really ease the symptoms.
Love
Ann

Here, probably the most significant action conducted is the offer of advice (*Das beste ist echt eine Therapie*), which implies (retrospectively) that Ann is treating Brenda's posting as a request for advice. If the advice implies that the first posting was a request (despite the fact that the first posting – not included in excerpt 9 – definitely did *not* contain a request), this suggests that Ann's posting as a whole is the second part of the "request – advice" adjacency pair. But the welcome, with which Ann opens her reply, is possibly also a second pair part of another adjacency pair. Therefore, we should not assume that only one action is being performed in postings.

Various factors in postings can indicate that the posting contains more than one action. In excerpt 9, for example, *Erstmal* (Firstly) is a marker of the performance of this action before the central or core action of the turn is produced. It signals that this posting contains at least two actions, and thus a label such as appreciation (in the case of Antaki et al., 2005) or advice fails to represent the welcoming action. A second aspect that implies that more than one action is performed is that some welcomes explicitly link it to an action produced by the first poster: An explanation of the courage it took to join HO. The overcoming of insecurity, articulated by novices in their first posting, is frequently lauded by the first recipient. Consider excerpts 10-13, which present excerpts 5-7 once again, but now including the first responses they received.

Excerpt 10 (#A2)

Veronika: N'abend…

So, nun trau ich mich auch mal  […]

Katja

Hallo Veronika,

[…]

Herzlich willkommen hier im Forum, schön daß du dich getraut hast zu schreiben![…]

Veronika: Evening…

So, now I'll also be brave  *[…]*

 # Katja: Hello Veronika,

[…]

A warm welcome to the forum, it's great that you were brave enough to write! […]

Excerpt 11 (#A17)

Martine: neu hier…

Hallo, angemeldet bin ich schon eine ganze Weile, aber erst habe ich nicht den Mut gefunden zu schreiben und dann ist die registrierung wieder in Vergessenheit geraten. Aber nun endlich…. Kurz zu mir: […]

Joe

hallallo martine

Herzlich willkommen hier im Forum, schön das du doch noch den mut gefunden hast etwas zu Posten, ich bin auch noch ziemlich neu hier im Forum und weiß auch noch das es auch lange gedauert hat bis ich was geschrieben habe wußte auch nicht so recht wie werde ich aufgenommen und so, aber ich kann dir sagen das du hier nur tolle Menschen findest und dir auch wirklich zuhören werden und dir auch helfen egal wie es einem gerade geht. […]

Martine: new here...

Hello,

I've been signed up already for quite a while, but I didn't find the courage to write at first and then the registration was forgotten. But now finally... About me: [...]

 # Joe:

hellello martine

A warm welcome to the forum, it's great that you did find the courage to post something, i'm also still relatively new to the forum and remember that it took a long time before i wrote something didn't really know how i would be accepted etc., but i can tell you that you will only find fantastic people here who will really listen to you and help you no matter how you're feeling at the time. [...]

Excerpt 12 (#A18)

Debby: ... bin ich essgestört?

Hallo zusammen! Vor einigen Tagen habe ich mich bei Euch im Forum angemeldet und nun sitze ich hier vorm PC und überlege, ob ich mich trauen soll, Euch als Aussenstehende die Frage zu stellen, ob ich eine Essstörung habe… wenn ich am Schluss den Beitrag abschicke, dann hab ich mich getraut… wir werden sehen.[…]

Louise

Hallo

Ich heiße Dich hier ganz herzlich Willkommen!

Der erste Schritt ist getan, dass Du Dich angemeldet und getraut hast, über Dich zu reden. Dass Schöne ist, dass Du hier ganz offen und ehrlich sein kannst, vor allen Dingen zu Dir selbst. Das hilft ungemein. Lanweilen tust Du niemanden, denn irgendwo sitzen wir alle im selben Boot, wir alle denken ständig über das Essen und unser Verhältnis dazu nach.[…]

Debby: ... do I have an eating disorder?
Hello everybody!
A few days ago I signed up with you in the forum and now I'm sitting here in front of the computer, thinking about whether I dare to ask you as outsiders whether I have an eating disorder... if I send off this post at the end, then I'll have dared... we'll see.
[...]
Now I've typed so much and will actually send it off now. I hope I won't bore anybody with it. [...]

 # Louise: Hello
A very warm welcome to you here!
The first step has been taken, that you've signed up and been brave enough to talk about yourself. The best thing is that you can be really open and honest here, above all to yourself. That helps enormously. You won't bore anybody because in some way we're all in the same boat, we all think constantly about food and our relationship to it. [...]

In excerpts 10-12, the recipients use exactly the same word (*trauen* or *Mut*) as the first poster did to express an appreciation of the fact that s/he has had the courage to contribute a posting. This implies that their insecurity is thus accepted as understandable or recognizable (most explicitly by Joe in excerpt 11, who mirrors the novice's initial lack of courage). In excerpts 10 and 11, this appreciation is packed into one sentence with a welcome to the forum, which articulates that these two actions (welcome and appreciation) are so close that they can occur in close proximity. [54]

In excerpt 13 (same as excerpt 1 plus first response), the word choice of the recipient is different from the novice's (*unsicher* vs. *getraut*), which suggests that the novice's insecurity exposed in the first posting can generally be read as requesting a welcome and some kind of appreciation as a second part.

---

[54] In the majority of cases, the insecurity is articulated in the beginning of the first posting, but even if it only appears at the end of the first posting, it still stimulates the respondent to offer a welcome and a show of appreciation.

Excerpt 13 (#33)

Antonia: Hallo bin neu…
Hallo ihr,
ich bin noch ein bisschen unsicher was ich hier schreiben soll. […]

Maggy
hallo
herzlich willkommen und schön dass du dich getraut hast hier zu schreiben. Du darfst
hier alles erzählen, alles was dich belastet […]

Antonia: Hello, I'm new…
Hello you guys,
I'm still a bit unsure about what I should write. […]

 # Maggie: hello
a warm welcome and it's great you were brave enough to write here. You can talk about anything here, anything that's troubling you […]

Here, again, the welcome and appreciation seem to be the second pair part of the insecurity.[55] Therefore, there is reason to argue that welcomes have a specific relationship to a first part, which could be that of an adjacency pair, but examining this in detail is impossible since the material is insufficient to detect "noticeable absence." We can only be certain of an adjacency pair, if it is observable when the second part is not produced (this is a consequence of its sequential relevance). This means that a welcome with appreciation would be observably absent when the first turn contains performed insecurity. Consider excerpt 14 (same as excerpt 2 plus first response), which represents the *only* case in the collection of threads in which the insecure opening did not receive a welcome with/without appreciation.

[55] The first pair part is not just the first posting as such, since there are also a number of cases in which the first posting does not display insecurity and does not receive a welcome. Hence, verbally marking a first posting as a first posting does not necessarily make a welcome with appreciation relevant. For instance, a posting which opens with *ich möchte mich erst einmal vorstellen bei euch* (I would first like to introduce myself to you), receives a very kind answer: *Das klingt ganz schön heftig* (That sounds pretty heavy), *not* followed by a welcome or explicit appreciation. These cases are evidence for the claim that particularly *insecure* first postings call up welcomes.

Excerpt 14 (#31)
Sylvia: bin ich gefährdet?
hallo ihr forumaner...
also eigentlich weiss ich gar nicht genau was ich hier schreiben soll [...]

Jennifer
Hallo,
ich habe Deinen Beitrag gelesen und dachte mir ich schreib dir mal. [...]

Sylvia: am I at risk?
hello you forumers...
so, i don't actually know what i should write here exactly [...]

 # Jennifer
Hello,
I read your post and thought I'd write back to you. [...]

Here, the response seems much less cordial compared to the welcomes and thus not quite offering reassurance to Sylvia's insecurity. Jennifer's opening expresses that Sylvia's first posting required an answer, but not necessarily a warm welcome. Thus, it suggests that the pair "insecurity – welcome" is a variant of the "request – compliance" adjacency pair, where the request concerns the wish to become a member of HO, and compliance is expressed by other members through the welcome. Adjacency pairs operate under a norm of preference (Pomerantz, 1984). The preferred second part to an offer is acceptance, the preferred second part of a greeting is a return greeting and the preferred second part of a request is compliance. For the present analysis, this implies that a welcome is the preferred response (= compliance) to a hesitant first posting, and the lack of a welcome the dispreferred alternative (= non-compliance). As the number of cases of this qualitative study is insufficient to examine the preference structure for insecure openings and welcomes more extensively, this aspect remains the subject for future investigation.[56]

What we can conclude at this point is that there is a strong tendency for an insecure first part to receive a welcome as a second part, but that this pattern may be disturbed when other actions within the first posting somehow constitute grounds to ignore the relevance of the second part. The character of turns

[56] A further question is why in some (but probably very few) cases, the preferred answer is not produced. For the thread of excerpt 14, the explanation is that after the insecure opening, Sylvia's first posting continues to be significantly different than those postings generally are. I will go into this "deviance" at length in chapter 8.

of asynchronous CMC (frequently consisting of many actions) makes it easier for something to thwart the production of the second pair part, which makes it potentially harder to recognize noticeable absence than in spoken interaction. Nevertheless, it could be that insecure beginnings form an adjacency pair with welcomes and appreciations. This does not imply that welcomes only occur in response to insecurity by the speaker in the prior turn.[57] However, if an insecure first posting does not receive a welcome, it *seems* at least noticeable absent.

6.6 Analysis: Identity and community accomplishment for settling membership

It was already argued that, during phone conversations, identities may be part of the situation in which the call takes place. First, I would like to propose a refinement of the concept of situational identity and second, I will consider a previous study of identity in a CMC forum opening.

The concept of situational identity has been argued to lack accuracy in openings and closings in phone calls to various Israeli radio shows (Hacohen, 2007). Hacohen found that different types of caller identities that are made relevant at the very beginning of the call appear to be consequential for the ensuing talk. The course of the interaction appears to vary depending on the acquaintance between caller and host. Hacohen identified various *local identities*, such as the standard caller, the first-time caller and the return caller, which are focused on at the beginning of the conversation. Let us have a look at some examples. (H = host and C = caller.)

The Standard Caller

H: Who would like to talk with Galey Zahal?

C: **Hello. Yitzhak is talking.**

H: Hello Yitzhak.

C: I wanted to say (continues)

---

[57] Welcomes likely form adjacency pairs with other actions as well. For instance, when a new member enters a group face-to-face, the welcome can be the first part and a thank you by the newcomer the second part. In fact, in HO, the novice members frequently also thank their recipient for the welcome. However, this does not seem to be related to insecurity.

The First Time Caller

H: Hallo? Hello?

C: Hello.

H: Hello Madam.

C: Yes. Ruth is speaking. I am Kibutznikit from Sha'ar HaNegev area.

H: Yes.

C: **I wanted- first of all, I ask you for a little help. It is the first time that I speak in a radio broadcast.**

H: **There is no problem, Ruth. I am all here for you.**

The Returning Caller

C: Good morning Gidon.

H: To you as well. What's your name.

H: Hello!

C: **My name is Haim Sapiriyan from Ramat HaGolan. For a long time I've not talked [to] you.**

H: How much is long time? […]

Source: Hacohen (2007: n.p.).

The First Time Caller could have made a standard call by just giving her name. But instead, she also produces her "first time" identity. Similarly, the Returning Caller could leave out his "return" identity and proceed as the Standard Caller does, but apparently, as the examples show, local identities are typically made relevant at the beginning of the conversation. Although the general situational identities are still intact (the host still acts as the host, and the caller remains the caller), Hacohen's cases demonstrate that the interaction achieves a refinement of situational identities to local identities, which are invoked by the participants themselves.

The concepts of situational and local identities are transferable to forum openings. The fact that a person posts a contribution in the New Here forum (being a poster) does not determine the local identity of the poster (being a novice member). For instance, the poster may not be a novice, or a novice member of a specific type, etc. Simultaneously, a novice member may "perform" actions that typically enact the poster identity, while not being related to the novice identity. Therefore, both situational and the more specific local identities should be taken into account.

Identities in online communities

Moving away from the beginnings of calls, a number of studies have focused on (group-) identity in (openings of) chat and forum conversations (e.g., Thimm and Ehmer, 2000; Benwell and Stokoe, 2006). Benwell and Stokoe's

(2006) analysis of a graphics chatroom reveals some general entry characteristics for a novice member to the community. Consider the following excerpt. (^_^ = "smiley face," *O_o* = "a nervous tick," *X_x* = "the writer is dead" [metaphorically].)

Irene:
Hey, I'm new and stuff^_^;
... And I suck at making topics like this
I've been lurking here a while now, and decided to finally
register ... I can't write fics that well but I love to read noir
shtuffs [*sic*]. Oh and I draw fanart. If you wanna call my crap art,
that is O_o
Now excuse me while I go chicken out here in the corner X_x

Browndog:
[EMOTICON]
Welcome! Oh, I'm the first one here! Coolness! SO you draw
do ya? That's great! But don't put yourself down! I'm sure
your art isn't as bad as you claim it is!
[...]
Have an Oreo and a devilled egg!
(not together, mind ya!) Welcome aboard and you better get a
vaccination for craziness because it spreads faster than wild fire
around here!
[...]

Source: Benwell and Stokoe (2006: 268).

The enactment of the situational identity of being novice in this thread was already pointed out in section 6.4. Furthermore, a welcome is here offered by the first recipient, quite similar to what was analyzed in section 6.5. Here, I would like to focus on identity and community work, which was observable in this particular CMC conversation.

Benwell and Stokoe argued that Irene not only performs the situational identity of newbie but also that of a regular, or expert member, namely through category-bound features, such as *making topics*, *writing fics*, *reading noir shtuffs* and *drawing fan art*. In doing so, however, she behaves self-deprecatingly, mitigating her own qualities: *I suck at making topics like this*, *I can't write fics that well*, etc. Benwell and Stokoe (2006: 274) explain that this self-deprecation is suggestive of a social order in which newbies lack status and must "earn" it from forum regulars who may be hostile. In other words, the situational identity of novice member may be related to a hierarchically lower position.

Irene is accepted as a new member through multiple and diverse acts in the two responses. The respondent performatively welcomes her (*Welcome!*), offers virtual gifts (*Have an Oreo and a devilled egg!*), uses colloquial language, give compliments (*SO you draw do ya? That's great!*), and uses humor (*a vaccination for craziness*). What the authors do not mention is that the welcome does not only perform Irene's acceptance, but also, constructs Browndog as a member who is in a position to welcome, and thus speak on behalf of the forum, and, in effect, it underscores Irene's novice identity. Browndog refers to the forum as a ship (*Welcome aboard*) and thus as a group, or community distinguishable from other communities.

Furthermore, I would like to emphasize the aspect of humor, which seems to have a special capacity. Irony is interwoven throughout the course of the thread, starting with some sentences in Irene's opening (*If you wanna call my crap art, that is O_o* and *Now excuse me while I go chicken out here in the corner X_x*), and thus irony appears to be a common way of soliciting solidarity. In other words, humor can be a community characteristic and, as such, can be used as a display of solidarity.

To summarize, various noticeable aspects that are observable in a thread analyzed by Benwell and Stokoe (2006) suggest general validity for online communities. Situational identities are attended to by participants of this piece of CMC interaction, and they are not restricted to the self, but also encompass doing another member's identity. Colloquial language use and humor may be used by a novice to "apply for" community membership and by regulars to articulate acceptance of the newbie.

Novices

The novice identity is frequently articulated as early as the subject line. Compare: *neu hier...* (#17) (new here), *Bin auch neu hier* (#23) (I am also new here), *Neu hier! BED?* (#25) (New here! BED?), *bin neu* (#27) (I am new), *Hallo bin neu...*(#33) (Hello I am new). However, a construction of the self as novice is not restricted to the initiator of the thread. Consider excerpt 15.

Excerpt 15 (#A8)

Monique: Erste Annäherung

[...]

#Angela
Hallo Monique,

ich bin zwar selber noch recht frisch hier, aber ich schreib dir gleich mal... HALLO!
[…] und mal ein Herzlich Willkommen von einer Neuen, an eine Neue… 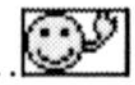

Monique: First approach
[...]

#Angela
Hello Monique,
I'm actually still really new here myself, but I'll write to you anyway... HELLO!
[...] and a Warm Welcome from one newcomer to another... 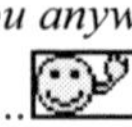

Angela's response to Monique in excerpt 15 demonstrates that, for a recipient who is still pretty new, the welcoming act requires an account. However, Angela still manages to perform a welcome twice and both times she emphasizes the shared novice status. Thus, Angela treats welcoming as something that is typically done by regulars or experts, and not by other novice members. At the same time, by welcoming Monique twice and the added emoticon, she seems very enthusiastic in the role of the welcomer. The reciprocity of being new at the same time offers camaraderie with the newbie's position.

Returners

There are many threads in the New Here forum that are not composed by novice members. Many returning members appear to re-enter the forum by composing a contribution to this sub-forum in particular. This identity of the one who is returning has frequently already been alluded to in the subject line: *wieder da* (#1) (here again), *wieder da und total am Ende* (#3) (here again and totally at the end), *hello again* (#13), *Neuer Versuch* (#14) (New attempt). This thus confirms Hacohen's distinction between various local identities for CMC forum interactions as well. I will explore one example (excerpt 16) in more detail.

Excerpt 16 (#A3)

Elena: wieder da und total am Ende
hi ihrz,
Weiss gar nicht wo ich das am besten hinschreibe…hoffe es passt einigermaßen. An-
sinsten sorry, einfach verschieben wo es besser passt.
Bin letztendlich wieder hier bei euch gelandet.[…]

Elena: here again and totally at the end
hi you guys,
Really don't know where would be best to write this…hope it's somewhat appropriate.
Otherwise sorry, just move it to a more suitable sub-forum.
Finally ended up here again with you. […]

Elena exhibits anxiety at the very beginning of her posting about the location of her posting, which may be inappropriate in both its content (*Weiss gar nicht* and *sorry*) and the ellipsis. Despite this uncertainty, she acts confidently (greeting and writing style are highly colloquial, she indexes the forum with a personal pronoun *euch*, she refers to "insider's knowledge" that moderators drag and drop postings to other sub-forums, etc.). The reason for the uncertainty is that this is a sub-forum for novice members and she is not new. She thus "orients to" the norm that says that the New Here sub-forum is intended for "real" newbies. This indicates that a novice identity is treated as the normative expectation. However, the excerpt demonstrates that one should not assume that all posters in this sub-forum are actually novices.

Representatives

It has already, with regard to excerpt 16, been suggested that welcoming is tied to a welcomer identity. I would like to argue that the activity of welcoming calls up the situational identity of "representative of the forum." Consider excerpt 17.

Excerpt 17 (#A2)
Veronika: N'abend…
[…]

Katja
Hallo Veronika,
[…] Herzlich willkommen hier im Forum, schön daß du dich getraut hast zu schreiben![…]

Veronika: Evening…
[…]

 # Katja: Hello Veronika,
[…] A warm welcome to the forum, it's great that you were brave enough to write!
[…]

We see here that *hier im Forum* is added to the welcome. Thus, Katja seems to speak on behalf of the whole forum. In other words, Katja identifies herself as a representative of the HO forum who fulfills the task of "officially" accepting a newcomer. Note that in face-to-face contexts, this role can only be played by those who have been legitimated to carry out this ritual. Hence, Katja's welcoming displays a distinction in status or position within HO: She implicitly ascribes Veronika the novice role, and adopts a representative, "official" role herself.

Community

First, I will demonstrate how community is discursively constructed by the participants and what is locally accomplished by this community constitution. While Benwell and Stokoe (2006) identified humor as one of the means to bolster solidarity between members, the initiation postings by novice members in HO and their responses seldom display humor or irony to create (a sense of) community. Irony may thus not be mistaken for a general CMC method used to establish solidarity in the community. Newbie's do not joke in HO, and regulars do not ironically welcome them. This finding suggests that other, "serious" strategies are operating in HO to produce community coherence.

Obviously the situational (and local) identities addressed above are also already bound to the community, which is the situation in which the interaction takes place (cf. Yates, 1996). However, the community is also explicitly articulated as a proper community. Consider Joe's response to Martine in excerpt 18 (same as the second part of excerpt 11 plus the next turn).

Excerpt 18 (#A17)

Martine: neu hier…
Joe
hallallo martine
Herzlich willkommen hier im Forum, schön das du doch noch den mut gefunden hast
etwas zu Posten, ich bin auch noch ziemlich neu hier im Forum und weiß auch noch
das es auch lange gedauert hat bis ich was geschrieben habe wußte auch nicht so recht
wie werde ich aufgenommen und so, aber ich kann dir sagen das du hier nur tolle
Menschen findest und dir auch wirklich zuhören werden und dir auch helfen egal wie
es einem gerade geht. […]

Martine (2)
Hallo Joe,

Danke fürs willkommen heißen. Ein paar nette Worte machen den einstieg doch etwas leichter.....
Liebe Grüße, martine

Martine: new here...
 # Joe
hellello martine
A warm welcome to the forum, it's great that you found the courage to post something, i'm also still relatively new to the forum and remember that it took a long time before i wrote something didn't really know whether i would be accepted etc., but i can tell you that you will only find fantastic people here who will really listen to you and help you no matter how you're feeling at the time. [...]

 # Martine (2)
Hello Joe,
Thanks for welcoming me. A few friendly words does make the initiation a bit easier.....
Love, martine

With regard to community, the verb *aufgenommen* (line 6) is essential. Generally speaking, being accepted or assimilated (= *aufgenommen*) is related to group membership. By using this verb, Joe treats HO as a community, as a group in which individuals can become accepted. Joe assures Martine that she will find only nice people in HO and thus implies that HO is a space of real people rather than just a board that merely offers individuals an opportunity to exchange information. Moreover, these members really listen (*wirklich zuhören*, line 7) rather than just read your posting and they even help regardless of how you are feeling at the time (*egal wie es einem gerade geht*, line 7). Thus, Joe suggests that HO members truly show their feelings, even if they are not doing so well.

What does this discursive production of HO as community accomplish? It serves to assure Martine that she is "safe" there, which she implicitly confirms by stating that Joe's words made her entrance or initiation (*einstieg*, line 12) easier. This implies that constructing HO as a community can operate as a reassuring detail for uncertain novice members. In spite of the assumption that this kind of interactional production of the HO forum co-constructs its being, Joe's construction of HO may not be considered as representative of how HO members experience HO participation.

The use of "doing" community as reassuring a hesitant, unconfident novice member is an action that is typically done by respondents. Novice members themselves, however, also use community as a tool to do interactional business, which seems to exhibit a more ambivalent stance towards HO as a community than when performed by respondents. Consider the exchange between Debby and Louise in excerpt 19 (same as excerpt 12).

Excerpt 19 (#A18)

Debby: .... bin ich essgestört?
Hallo zusammen! Vor einigen Tagen habe ich mich bei Euch im Forum angemeldet
und nun sitze ich hier vorm PC und überlege, ob ich mich trauen soll, Euch als Au-
ssenstehende die Frage zu stellen, ob ich eine Essstörung habe… wenn ich am Schluss
den Beitrag abschicke, dann hab ich mich getraut… wir werden sehen. […]

Louise
Hallo
Ich heiße Dich hier ganz herzlich Willkommen!
Der erste Schritt ist getan, dass Du Dich angemeldet und getraut hast, über Dich zu
reden. Dass Schöne ist, dass Du hier ganz offen und ehrlich sein kannst, vor allen
Dingen zu Dir selbst.
Das hilft ungemein.
Lanweilen tust Du niemanden, denn irgendwo sitzen wir alle im selben Boot, wir alle
denken ständig über das Essen und unser Verhältnis dazu nach. […]

Debby: ... do I have an eating disorder?
Hello everybody!
A few days ago I signed up with you in the forum and now I'm sitting here in front of the computer, thinking about whether I dare to ask you as outsiders, whether I have an eating disorder... if I send off the post at the end, then I'll have dared... we'll see. [...]

 # Louise: Hello
A very warm welcome to you here!
The first step has been taken, that you've signed up and been brave enough to talk about yourself. The best thing is that you can be really open and honest here, above all to yourself. That helps enormously. You won't bore anybody because in some way we're all in the same boat, we all think constantly about food and our relationship to it. [...]

Starting from the greeting, Debby "orients to" a community by explicitly addressing the "togetherness" of her readers. Although *bei Euch im Forum* (line 1) displays a similar invocation of a community, *Euch als Aussenstehende* (line 2) does more than merely refer to a group. It emphasizes the boundary between an inside (Debby) and an outside (HO), addressing the HO members as outsiders.[58] Debby is a new member, so why would she emphasize that she does not belong to the community? The subject line offers an explanation. Since Debby is not certain that she is actually eating disordered, she cannot directly see herself as part of the community. In other words, she enacts a local identity as novice member, which is not necessarily an "application" to be accepted as a "real" member. Note that local identity (being novice) and categorical identity (being eating disordered or not) occur simultaneously, and may even conflict in the interaction. The community is in this way used both to apply for membership and to distance herself from the community.

Louise's reply is a very subtle answer to Debby's question of whether she is eating disordered (congruent with the adjacency pair of question and answer), and uses the *community* to tailor this answer. Louise performs the welcoming act very warmly and refers to Debby's posting as the first step, which is specified as having registered and having had the courage to talk about herself. So far, she has treated Debby as a novice member who has been accepted in HO, avoiding a re-construction of HO members as outsiders. This is the first step in providing an answer: If Debby is accepted into the community, she may share the identity of "being eating disordered" with the other members.

Louise then goes one step further: *Das Schöne ist, dass Du hier ganz offen und ehrlich sein kannst, vor allen Dingen zu Dir selbst* (line 10-11) The good thing (*das Schöne*) is not that you finally have someone to tell all your problems to (cf. Joe's sense of community), but, more importantly, you can be open and honest to yourself in the forum. Put differently, HO is not defined as a medium to communicate with *others*, but primarily with *oneself*. As an answer to Debby's question, this means that Louise is advising Debby to admit to herself that she is eating disordered. In other words, a definition of HO is given *as* an answer to the question of whether Debby is eating disordered: You can be open and honest to yourself. Hence, the reference to HO as a community is not simply used to make Debby feel safe, but to tell her what to do. Line 12 supports the value of this advice: It is an extraordinary help. "It" refers to being open and honest to yourself, and thus indirectly also admitting that you have an eating problem, or an affirmative answer to the question posed in the subject line. (The issue of admitting the eating disorder is further discussed in chapter 8.)

The continuation of Louise's reply can be seen as an invocation of community to convey safety and belonging (as Joe's was in reply to Martine in excerpt 19). Louise assures Debby that she is not boring anyone, *denn irgendwo sitzen wir alle im selben Boot* (line 13). The idiomatic expression "being in

---

[58] This is striking because the community is usually portrayed as the in-group, and the novice member as the outsider.

the same boat" obviously means that all HO members have something, namely a specific type of problem, in common. The response to Debby's opening lines 1-4, which uses this saying, again blurs the boundary between Debby and HO outsiders, and includes Debby in HO. In other words, a virtual community construction again works interactionally to express that Debby is one of them (*Der erste Schritt is getan, dass Du Dich angemeldet und getraut hast, über Dich zu reden*, line 9), but also in terms of sharing the same problems (*irgendwo sitzen wir alle im selben Boot*, line 12). Hence, reference to HO as a community operates as a bridge between the individual and the collective of eating disorder sufferers. But being in the same boat also implies that HO members are a group of victims. Louise does not write that HO members have eating problems as such in common, but she points out that they are all constantly thinking about food and their relation to it: *wir alle denken ständig über das Essen und unser Verhältnis dazu nach* (line 13-14). Only the word *ständig* implies that this thinking is problematic. The interactional use of it is that Louise avoids directly speaking of the HO community as a group of ill people, and thus mitigates the inclusion of Debby as one of them. The community that is grounded on something that is shared, which does not overtly imply being ill, allows Louise to avoid declaring that she considers Debby to be ill (which would be face-threatening).

The interaction between Debby and Louise reveals that community membership for certain novices is controversial. Debby clearly positions herself outside of the community in her opening, while Louise explicitly treats Debby as one of them.

6.7 Conclusion

During the first interactional steps in HO by the novice member, the community and various identities are deployed and established in numerous ways. Novice members are hesitant and uncertain, at least during the initiation phase into HO. HO novices seem to display a more extensive or more profound degree of caution than newbies generally do (cf. Benwell and Stokoe, 2006). Thus, the analysis of openings suggests that entering the HO forum is difficult. Returning members display less insecurity than "real" novices.

Respondents routinely welcome the novice member using a kind of formula, which may not be typical of HO, but of newsgroup/mailinglist/ forum conversation in general (cf. Thimm and Ehmer, 2000). For the regulars that do the welcoming, it has been shown that the performance of this act can mean assuming responsibility for the novice, while simultaneously positioning themselves as representatives and the novice as new.

The question is what this "official" welcoming does for the hesitant novice. On the one hand, it may give her/him the feeling of acceptance, which can certainly alleviate the burden of joining. On the other hand – although this is speculation – it could also be part of why it is difficult to join HO, and why it requires courage. The ritualistic welcome means being assimilated, and that is exactly what some novice members have been ambivalent about (excerpt 19). What if you do not know whether you really have an eating disorder or not or you do not want to admit it? In these cases, it may seem "undesirable" or even threatening to be officially welcomed and accepted as a member. These are thoughts that are developed in detail in subsequent chapters. However, the openings and the responses already indicate that joining HO is a multilayered process that is negotiated or, better yet, accomplished through interaction. Since some novice members clearly indicate that they are unsure of whether they have actually knocked on the right door, entering HO as a novice member can best be described as a sensitive task, while welcoming is an important task for the regulars to accommodate the novice and offer advice.

Chapter 7

Displaying forumability in the online community

7.1 Introduction

After having commenced with their first posting with some hesitance, novice members describe the types of eating problems they are struggling with. In presenting this description, a person is simultaneously engaged in a presentation of self (Heritage and Robinson, 2006: 48). This perspective on identity, which is acted out in conversation mainly through the use of categories, is central to this chapter. Another important point of entry is that it has been found that, in various types of settings, asking for help is an "accountable" activity (e.g., Edwards and Stokoe, 2007; Heritage and Robinson, 2006; Whalen and Zimmerman, 1990). In fact, displaying accountability is a normative requirement not only for institutional settings:

> There is a particular accountability in asking for help in cases in which it is not immediately obvious that the requester is unable to solve the problem themselves, or ... in which one is consulting strangers or experts on personal matters when one might be expected to turn first to friends and family (Edwards and Stokoe, 2007: 10).

In this chapter, I demonstrate that participants display accountability when they join the HO forum. This accountability, in the context of the HO forum, can concretely be described as the concern for *forumability*, which establishes whether a given problem is appropriate to the available service. In cases of accountability, we expect that various normative requirements will play a role in how participants present themselves or their problems. I focus here on whether and how identity categories are relevant to felicitous accounting in becoming a HO member. It appears that the HO's expectations or normative requirements include the preliminary intention of seeking self-help, which means that HO members construct appropriate behavior that makes them not seem to be dependent on the services HO offers.

Other requirements concern projecting onself as eating disordered (since considerate time, usually years), preferably through diagnoses in the form of abbreviations (section 7.4 and 7.5). This type of self-presentation generally elicits acts of acceptance by other members through reciprocal self-presentations (section 7.6). Subtle levels of friction or tension can be observed during certain interactions when the novice does not yet have a clear diagnosis (section

7.7), or does not fully recognize the severity of her/his problem (section 7.9), but this does not necessarily mean that the novice is indirectly rejected by HO. (More serious threats to forumability are closely analyzed in chapter 8). Problematic orientations are also found when the novice not only has eating disorders, but multiple psychic disorders such as borderline, depression and self-inflictive behavior (section 7.8), or when s/he is older than the presumed age for those with eating disorders (after adolescence) (section 7.10). These potential problems are, however, defused by the respondents, who indirectly confirm that these particular issues are unusual or problematic, but also express the notion that these issues do not jeopardize the members' forumability.

Another point I will address is the notion that forumability is closely linked to being a community. The normative requirements that participants "orient to" and articulate in their accounts are co-constitutive of the community, especially when not only the novice's accounts but recipients' responses to these accounts are also considered. In this respect, forumability is expressing accountability for the membership of a unique community.

7.2 Forumability: A matter of accountability and identity

Generally, accounts are descriptions that name, characterize, formulate, explain, excuse, excoriate, or merely take notice of some circumstance or activity and thus place it within some social framework (West and Zimmerman, 1987:136). Focusing on turns in an interaction, accountability thus refers to how

> actors design their actions in relation to their circumstances so as to permit others, by methodically taking account of circumstances, to recognize the action for what it is (Heritage, 1984: 179).

Thus, actors are held accountable for *which* action they conducted. However, a more specific form of accountability is that actors can be confronted with the question of *why* they conducted this action. I focus on this extensive understanding of accountability. In previous research on medical interactions, this type of accountability was encountered. When patients seek medical care, they present their problems in such a way that the physician becomes the right person to consult. They frequently use accounts to do this. Heritage and Robinson (2006) demonstrated how patients account for the medical visit in the course of their interaction with a physician. The main premise in Heritage and Robinson's analysis was that patients, by walking into a physician's office, commit themselves to the belief that they have a legitimate reason for coming. Put differently, patients design their description of events, experiences and circumstances to communicate "good reasons" that will justify their making an appointment. This is why it is patients' task to present their medical problems as *doctorable* (Heritage and Robinson, 2006).[59]

Forumability

An attempt to translate doctorability to the online setting of a health support forum would be to presume that the novice member should present (herself/himself with) her/his problems as *forumable*. However, this juxtaposition requires some reflection. Presenting problems as forumable is different from presenting them as doctorable. The settings and participants of the situation in which the problems are presented are notably dissimilar. The HO forum as a textual space cannot be equated with the physician's office and the HO participants are not a (team of) physician(s). For instance, we cannot assume that a novice member will consider the other forum participants as entitled to make a diagnosis, which is precisely what a patient can assume about a physician's competence. It could be that HO-forum participants display similar concerns as they would in a physician's office, but we cannot assume this. Furthermore, although the means of communication do not intrinsically *determine* the interactional mechanisms, an analysis must at least be attentive to the relations between channels and contents. Whereas a presentation of the problem at the physician's office can be accounted for by demonstrating bodily deficiency, the online visit lacks this channel of interaction. These considerations indicate that the term forumable can only be understood *after* a study of how novice members present themselves and their problems in this forum, and not as a presupposition. Nevertheless, the concern for forumability has opened our eyes to practices in web-based, health support forums that are potentially similar to those in the physician's office.

Previous studies have revealed numerous features of accountability and help seeking. In mediation requests for disputes between neighbors it has been discovered that a normative preliminary act is that the complainer has already tried to speak to the complained-of neighbor (Edwards and Stokoe, 2007). In a physician's office patients justify their visit by 1) making diagnostic claims, 2) invoking third parties as the ones who persuaded them to go see the doctor, and 3) making "trouble resistant" claims (Heritage and Robinson, 2006). These trouble resistant claims can be explained by Parsons' (1951) assumption that people labor under the obligation to resist the *sick role*. Although

[59] The term *doctorability* is derived from *policeability* (Meehan, 1989). These concepts can generally be described as features of service provision, which establish that a given problem is appropriate for the service being requested (Edwards and Stokoe, 2007).

going to the physician is already a sign of one's weakening resistance, patients still exhibit "trouble resistance" during the medical consultation process. They may reveal that they have tried to cope with the problem on their own prior to seeking medical care or they may express that they are currently coping with their problems. In this way, the problem is presented in an objective "just the facts" approach, which is a sign of trouble resistance. Furthermore, trouble resistance was observed in calls for professional help at a suicide help line. These calls seem to be accounted for by treating the help line as a last resort rather than the first person turned to (Sacks, 1972).

These features are indirectly related to the identity of the help-seeker, since being ill, being suicidal, as well as having trouble with one's neighbor, can be expected as a pre-condition for the initial step of calling or visiting a doctor, or posting on a forum in the first place. Presenting the self as having a problem is thus an account; it can be done by, for instance, presenting the self as eating disordered, suicidal, depressed, an alcoholic, etc.

Consequentiality of identity categories

In analyzing the co-occurrence of accountability and identity (categories), it is important to scrutinize the consequentiality of categories in interaction, since categories are not necessarily sequentially relevant. I will illustrate this by pointing to a study by Edwards (1998). He analyzed the first counseling session of Connie and Jimmy, a couple with marital problems. The presentation of relevant categories is here initiated by the therapist, and not by Connie and Jimmy themselves. Early in the session, the therapist elicits identity categorizations "that presumably have some relevance to the business at hand, such as (generally speaking) relationship trouble and counseling" (Edwards, 1998: 18).

Counsellor:	[...] hh how old are you now?
Connie:	I'm thirty fi:ve,
	(0.6)
Jimmy:	Thirty five.
	(0.4)
Counsellor:	Right. And you've been married how many years
Connie:	Just twelve years now
Jimmy:	Thirteen years [in September]
Connie:	[Thirteen years] in September

Source: Edwards (1998: 19). The original transcript is radically simplified by me.

Edwards suggests that the details the therapist requests, although seemingly routine (demographic), already suggest "what *kinds* of 'sense' they *may* provide" (Edwards, 1998: 22, emphasis in original). For instance, in the excerpt above, age may add an extra context to the marital problems. Connie's and Jimmy's ages could be a potential basis to help explain shared or incompatible interests, expectations, and/or types of relationships and thus it could explain their marital problems. However, CA principles do not permit the use of this kind of tacit knowledge regarding categories like age in the analysis. Instead,

> the analytic[al] task is not to produce idealized and presumptive stories of this kind, nor to use them as a 'given' basis for analysts' explanations, or psychological models, of what people do or say. Our task is to examine what it is, if anything, that people do with these categorizations (Edwards, 1998: 23).

In Edwards' analysis, the category of age was not discovered to be relevant, possibly because Connie and Jimmy were about the same age and thus it was not considered a "rhetorical" resource for them to discuss their problems. However, the identity as a married woman did seem to be relevant.

> Connie: ...normally as I said it's either maybe somebody's birthday. (0.2) That's a reason we go out an' have a few drinks, another it could be: somebody has a problem like recently a friend of mine had a problem that wanted to talk, these are the nights out, these are the things we sit around one table full of married women, (0.2) an that's normally our nights out ...

Source: Edwards (1998: 30). The original transcript is radically simplified by me.

For the purpose of distinguishing her night out from Jimmy's, Connie establishes herself as a member of a group of married women by describing category-bound features of the "normal" kind of a night out for this group (celebrating a birthday, talking about problems, sitting around a table). She does not use the category "married women" here simply because that is what she is. Instead, she uses this category at this specific moment in the interview to counter Jimmy's allegation that she also has her "girls' nights out." The excerpt illustrates that categorization can locate someone as a member of one group or another and that group membership can be invoked and deployed for local, "personal" business. This is what people attend to in their conversations. While age was not a consequential identity here, gender was. Hence, the interrelation of identity and accountability cannot be presumed, but must be shown to be made relevant by the participants.

Illness identity as display of forumability

As argued above, a description of (having) an illness can be a way to justify the seeking of help. In a US online support forum on depression, members appeared to introduce themselves as depressed but nevertheless competent people (Lamerichs, 2003). Since the relevant concept here, as in HO, can be argued to be forumability, I will consider some of Lamerichs' excerpts.[60] The central question is how participants present themselves as forumable. I will show that, in this particular forum, forumability encompasses being not too severely depressed and being knowledgeable of the various medical/diagnostic terms. Consider Diana's first posting on the forum.

> Diana: Thanks for opening up this folder. I am bi-polar (manic-depressive) of the not too severe type. The depression part has been in my family for generations as well as agoraphobia, (myself, my mother and grandmother), panic disorder (mother, grandmother and daughter). I believe the theory that it can be genetic. I also believe that hormones play a huge part in it ...

Source: Lamerichs (2003: 83).

Lamerichs notes that Diana presents her depression as an accountable matter, and that the actual account is externalized responsibility: Her depression is genetic/biological. Obviously, this also implies that presenting yourself as depressed is a way of presenting yourself as forumable. Lamerichs argues that Diana's presentation of herself in this line is an illustration of the fact that she is pointing out the reason why she came to the forum in the first place. Seemingly, Lamerichs induces that being depressed is a legitimate and sufficient reason for joining the forum.

However, the *way* that Diana presents herself as depressed is rather specific and could be more specifically related to forumability. Let us have a closer look at the sentence: *I am bi-polar (manic-depressive) of the not too severe type*. The use of the medical diagnostic term "bi-polar" exhibits knowledgeability of diagnostic vocabulary, supplemented by a display of awareness that this medical term may not be understood by everyone: *(manic-depressive)*. Subsequently she adds *of the not too severe type*, which counters the image of a hopelessly depressed person. Hence, besides presenting herself as depressed and not responsible for her condition, she constructs herself as a knowledgeable and not too severely depressed person. She receives the following response:

[60] Lamerichs (2003) herself did not consider forumability, but, instead, focused on depression as an accountable matter. Despite this difference in analytical scope, the material does give some interesting cues that could be related to forumability.

Liz: I too am glad to see this topic being discussed. I am a psychologist and I have been treated for depression. Sometimes depression runs in families and it doesn't need an event triggering it ...

Source: Lamerichs (2003: 83).

Liz first presents herself as a psychologist and thereafter as having been treated for depression. What does a presentation of "being a psychologist" accomplish? Given that this forum is an online support forum, the participants' professional identity may at first be regarded as irrelevant. For Liz, however, it is relevant. The category psychologist infers category-bound features such as "knowing diagnostic vocabulary," which was also displayed in Diana's first posting. It also allows her to make a statement about the epidemiology of depression, such as: *Sometimes depression runs in families and it doesn't need an event triggering it.* Her orientation to her professional identity is thus an alignment with Diana's self presentation: Both are able to discuss depression in medical terminology. Furthermore, Liz mitigates her own "disordered" identity by describing herself as having *been treated for depression*, which leaves her current condition open. Locally however, it allows her to enact a personal experience with depression, without presenting herself as solely a sufferer. The fact that, in the design of the turn, the professional category is prioritized to the disordered identity suggests that being knowledgeable about depression is more relevant in this particular situation than being experienced as a sufferer of depression.

Another example from Lamerichs' study exhibits further sensitivity not only to the external causes of depression (*depression "for a reason"*), but also to the current state of the disorder and medical terminology.

Dorothy: I am pleased to see this folder come into existence. I had experienced depression brought on by working hard to get a college degree, while juggling a household with three children, and then being unable to get a job... That's depression "for a reason" – I think there is a double barreled psychological term for it, but I can't remember what it is. That depression disappeared as soon as I did land a job! Then, there is the current situation – not depression, but being "at risk for".

Source: Lamerichs (2003: 82).

Not unlike Diana, Dorothy also does not present herself as actually suffering severely from depression. In fact, the examples of introductions of novice members that Lamerichs presents all mitigate the actual seriousness of the problem (e.g., "previously depressed" or "not severely depressed"). This is not to say that in this online support forum participants never exhibit the deep down feelings of depression; however, they do not seem to do so in their first postings. Furthermore, Dorothy also presents relevant diagnostic information by referring to a psychological term, which she used to know, but does not recall at the moment she is typing her posting. The orientation to the psychological term, despite the fact that she cannot remember it, is an indication of its relevance.

Naturally, the few contributions that I have considered here are insufficient to draw any conclusion on forumability in this particular online support forum on depression. Nonetheless, the excerpts provided by Lamerichs suggest that forumability in that setting includes being not too severely depressed, and being fairly knowledgeable of medical/diagnostic terms. This raises the question of whether this is characteristic of a forum dealing with depression, or whether this is also the case for a forum on eating disorders, or even characteristic of online communities in general. To compare, Benwell and Stokoe (2006) contended that in online environments, colloquial language use (e.g., words like *suck*, *crap*, *chicken out*) operates to bolster one's solidarity with other members. This suggests that generalizations about the way to display forumability are doubtful. In some forums, a fashion to display one's forumability is colloquial language use, whereas, in other forums, it is the use of professional (medical) terminology.

Characteristic features of forumability can be compared to what is found in other settings of service provision. Heritage and Robinson (2006), for instance, demonstrate how patients use diagnostic claims at a physician's office. These may be sanctioned or challenged by the doctor, but self-diagnosis can also be a trump card in claiming doctorability, for example, in cases where a patient has experience with a particular problem. Moreover, the feature of presenting the self as not too severely depressed is similarly observed in medical interactions, where trouble resistance displays the patient as able to cope, and as self-managing (Heritage and Robinson, 2006). In contrast, Edwards and Stokoe (2007) found that callers frequently use extreme case formulations (Pomerantz, 1986) when they recount the problems they have experienced with their neighbors. That is to say, in this service setting, asking for help is not accompanied by claims of being able to cope, but, instead, justified by sketching the problem as extreme.

These cursory comparisons indicate that accounting for one's behavior may be done in distinct fashions in different settings. Lamerichs and Te Molder (2003) are implicit about the relation between the situation (or setting) of the online forum on depression and the interaction that is taking place. They suggest that "part of the identity work may be related to the mental health setting" (Lamerichs and Te Molder, 2003: 469). This chapter takes up this question and will try to come to a more precise description of the relation between the forum setting and the role identity (work) plays in it.

7.3 Goal and method

This part of the analysis of HO postings attempts to come to terms with how members justify their joining HO, i.e., how they deal with the issue of forumability in the first interactions, and to understand the role of identity in these accounts. The interaction with recipient HO members is crucial here, since, in their responses, they may either accept or decline the offered account and/or propose other possible accounts. Questions that informed the analysis included: Do members explicitly offer accounts for their online visits? What is considered a legitimate account? To what extent are accounts delivered in terms of identity? What do these presentations of identity look like? Which self-presentations are treated as forumable by the recipients?

With regard to the analytical concepts of identity and community, the concept categorical identity and situational identity (Zimmerman, 1998) are used not only as distinct concepts, but additionally as potentially co-constructive, i.e., a categorical identity can go together with and occasion a situational identity and vice versa. Moreover, the analysis presented in this chapter draws on the concept and theory of Membership Categorization Devices (Schegloff, 2007). An analysis of how categories are used in naturally occurring interactions, so-called Membership Categorization Analysis (MCA) is "concerned with the organisation of common-sense knowledge in terms of the categories members employ in accomplishing their activities in and through talk" (Francis and Hester, 2004:21). Several characteristics of categories of talk were already introduced in chapter 1.2, among which category-bound activities (categories and members of categories are linked to particular actions) and inference richness. Additionally, MCA supposes that categories follow certain rules of application, which are (unconsciously) known by speakers and these are thus important to observe for the present analysis.

The "economy rule" holds that a single category from any Membership Category Device can in principle do adequate reference (for instance "a ballerina"). However, more *can* be used (for instance "45-year-old Russian ballerina"). Schegloff has linked the observation that in principle one term *can* do adequate reference to the analysts' task of hermeneutic interpretation in actual cases in which more than one category is used: "If one reference can be enough, why wasn't it?" (2007: 471). Another rule is the "consistency rule," which, for instance, states that if several people have to categorize themselves, the category collection picked up by the first speaker can be used by the subsequent speaker. So, if a person introduces her/himself as a 30-year-old, s/he makes the category collection of *age* relevant for the next person to introduce her/himself, instead of, for instance, the collections of profession, nationality or illness. Schegloff (2007: 471) has stressed, however, that this is an optional practice, rather than a mandatory one.

Presenting the self is an instance of doing identity. But, presenting the self reciprocally is also a means to display acceptance of the novice member and thereby offering community membership. These aspects are not focused here, since they reflect a lot of what has been spelled out in chapter 2.3. Nonetheless, they are touched upon along the way, since they do form one of the central themes of the study.

Note that:

- Nicknames are replaced by pseudonyms, and age is replaced by age groups for the sake of anonymity.
- Text inside brackets in the excerpts is either anonymized information added by the author (W.S) or the description of an emoticon/smiley.
- The excerpt codes (#...) refer to the unique position of data in the data set.
- The typing, spelling and punctuation are original.
- The English translations of postings are added for the sake of comprehension, but the original German messages are the actual research material.

7.4 Analysis: Overt displays of forumability

At first sight, a very common way to introduce oneself to the other forum members is a presentation in terms of at least two features: Age[61] and eating disorder, including the duration of the eating disorder. The role of such presentations of the self regarding accountability is investigated here. The analyses offer a detailed tracking of what these categories do in the HO interaction. First, however, overt formulations of one's justification for joining the forum are analyzed. I will examine whether novice members explicitly account for their joining the forum. As argued above, though related to (mental) health issues, we cannot simply assume that someone's reason for joining HO is generally "seeking medical care" as it would for someone going to a doctor. In the rare cases in which reasons for joining are explained, they are usually preceded by a presentation of the self in terms of age, type of eating disorder, and the history of the disorder.

It appears that novice members rarely deliver literal accounts for their joining the forum such as "I am here, because...," which suggests that one is not required to *overtly* account for one's participation in HO. However, some nov-

[61] For ethical reasons, participants' ages are substituted by an age group. These are: <18, 18-22, 23-30, 31-35 and 35-40.

ice members do produce accounts for joining and/or they further indicate what they imagine the forum might be useful for. In this section, I will demonstrate that some overt accounts for joining HO are similar to general accounts for seeking help, while others are rather dissimilar. The self-help preliminary intention and the invocation of third parties are similar, but what is surprising are the trouble-resistant claims that enable these novice members to avoid explicit help requests. Instead, they display self-responsibility for their recovery and thus suggest that they do not expect the forum to solve their problems. Thus, members "orient to" HO as an ambiguous entity: On the one hand, it is treated as a help service, while, on the other hand, joining HO is not constructed as "the last resort" type of help-service. Instead, participants suggest, for instance, that it is only a form of support to deal with the problem alone (hence, just a small step on the long way to recovery). In excerpt 1, this ambiguity is readily observed.

Excerpt 1 (#21)

Wendy: hallo alle miteinander

[...]

Es ist ein Auf und ein Ab und ich bin jetzt zum Schluss gekommen, dass ich mir helfen lassen muss, dass ich es nicht alleine schaffe. Der erste Schritt war, mich hier anzumelden. Ich möchte kämpfen, möchte meine Essstörung in den Griff bekommen, die zurzeit leider mich im Griff hat. Ich finde es klasse, dass es solche Foren wie dieses hier gibt. Danke dafür.

LG [nickname]

Wendy: hello everybody

[...]

I've been going back and forth, and I've now come to the conclusion that I have to get some help, that I can't do it alone. The first step was to register here. I want to fight, want to get a grip on my eating disorder, which unfortunately has a grip on me at the moment. I think it's great that there are forums like this. Thank you for that.

Love [nickname]

Wendy realizes that she needs to seek help because she is not able to manage all by herself. This is similar to the account that *one cannot help oneself*, or the preliminary norm of self-help (Edwards and Stokoe, 2007; Sacks, 1972). However, the insight that she needs help is not formulated as a request for help. Wendy mainly equates the *first* step of recovery with registering for the forum. She does not specify what she expects from the forum, but the determined *ich möchte kämpfen* (line 4) implies that she is not passively waiting for the forum to solve her problems. While a doctor may offer a solution to a medical problem, Wendy points out that *she* wants to get her eating disorder under control herself. In other words, the account avoids asking for other people's help and focuses on self-help. Hence, justifying joining HO has a contradictory effect. On the one hand, the novice admits that she cannot cope alone, but, on the other hand, she resists asking for help in the sense that she emphasizes that she will try to get a grip on the problem by herself. The forum is thus constructed as the medium between the self and self-help or a help-service for people who seek self-help. In excerpt 2, Martine displays how she manages alone, which means she is not urgently in need of help.

Excerpt 2 (#17)

Martine: neu hier…

[…]

Eigentlich kann ich mich überhaupt nicht daran erinnern, jemals ein normales, ausgeglichenes Essverhalten gehabt zu haben. Seit ein paar Monaten Lebe ich nun weitgehens ohne Fressen und kotzen, denke aber, dass die Möglichkeit, gelegentlich sich auszutauschen, hilfreich wäre, dass es auch so bleibt. Darum hab ich mich entschlossen, nun doch zu schreiben. […]

Martine: new here…

[…]

Actually, I can't remember ever having had a normal, balanced relationship to food. I've been living for a few months now mostly without binging and purging, but think that the possibility of comparing notes occasionally would be helpful in keeping it that way. That's why I've decided that I will actually write now. […]

Martine makes a so-called trouble resistant claim as her reason for joining the HO forum, indicated by the word *darum* in line 5. She presents herself as mostly (*weitgehens*, line 3) managing on her own (referring to binging and vomiting). This claim can be delivered to counter the idea that Martine would immediately consult strangers regarding a personal problem, her eating disorder. In fact, she is coping on her own, but the opportunity to occasionally engage in dialogue would be helpful (line 4-5). In other words, here exchange in the HO forum is not constructed as the *first* step out of the disorder, but as one step in a progressive recovery process. It reduces the help question to a last push or a little support in the process of self-help.

Third parties are frequently alluded to in help-seeking discourses. Heritage and Robinson (2006: 71) have demonstrated that in doctor-patient interactions, *third parties*, i.e., notable others such as partners, relatives, and friends, are invoked to support a patient's accounts for arranging a visit. First, the patient's problems, which lead to the decision to see the doctor, are already validated by another person and second, the responsibility for seeking medical attention is reduced or attenuated. In first postings to the HO forum, third parties are also invoked, but not necessarily as "validators." In excerpt 3, the third party is staged as unable to help. The invocation of a third party therefore seems to support the claim that the novice has "no one to turn to," but this is only true because the novice member is *unable* to ask for help. Becoming a member of HO is thus treated as a triumph over this inability. Consider excerpt 3.

Excerpt 3 (#8)

Monique: Erste Annäherung

[...]

Vor drei Jahren ungefähr fing dann die Bulimie an, lange Zeit nur selten, jetzt kommen die Attacken jedoch immer öfter und ich bemerke, dass ich alleine es nicht schaffe. Ich weiß, dass die Einsicht der erste Schritt ist, allerdings hat sie mich vor erneuten Fressattacken bis jetzt nur selten bewahrt. Deswegen würde ich gerne mit Menschen in kontakt treten, die ähnliche Probleme haben und die mir, so hoffe ich, ein wenig helfen können. Hier habe ich nämlich keinen, weil ich es einfach nicht schaffe, jemanden um Hilfe zu bitten. Meinem Freund habe ich es vor etwa einem Jahr gesagt, allerdings ist er auch machtlos, will mir helfen, weiß aber nicht wie. Ich habe mich auch immer vor diesem Thema verschlossen. Jetzt hoffe ich, dass ich durch diesen Schritt ein wenig offener werde, auch gegenüber Menschen, die ich in meiner Nähe habe. [...]

Monique: First approach

[...]

Then about three years ago, the bulimia began, for a long time only rarely, but the attacks are happening more and more often now, and I realize that I can't deal with it alone. I know that recognition is the first step, although until now this has rarely prevented renewed bouts of binging. That's why I would like to get in touch with people who have similar problems, and who I hope can help me a little. That is, I don't have anyone here, because I simply can't manage to ask anybody for help. I told my boyfriend about a year ago, but he is also helpless, wants to help me, but doesn't know how. I've also always denied this topic to myself. Now I hope this step will help me to be a bit more open, also to the people around me.

[...]

In line 5, the delivered accounts for joining are marked with the word *deswegen*. First, the account of not being able to help oneself is again stated (line 3). Unlike Wendy in excerpt 1, Monique distinguishes between the first step as recognition of the inability to cope by oneself and the subsequent step of joining HO. She further accounts for her seeking help in HO by invoking a third party as a reason for joining: Her boyfriend. He is not invoked as a validator of the problem, but as one of the reasons she is joining HO, because he is unable to offer support or help (line 7-9). This account is thus the indirect recognition of the normative expectation that when someone has personal problems, one should first turn to friends and family. Logically, when someone claims that these people cannot help, it offers one the excuse or reason to seek help elsewhere.

A similar phenomenon has been described in detail by Sacks (1972), in which a caller to a suicide help line claims: *I have no one to turn to*. Sacks explains this by showing that the normative expectation is that one should ask intimates for help before turning to a professional help service, in other words, that professional help is a last resort. Monique's account starts similarly (*Hier habe ich nämlich keinen*, line 6-7), but continues in a significantly different vein: Because I simply cannot manage to ask anybody for help *(weil ich es einfach nicht schaffe, jemanden um Hilfe zu bitten*, line 7). Her boyfriend seems to be the exception: She told *him* a year ago, and he is willing to help, but is unable to do so. Hence, she has no one to turn to, because she is unable to ask for help. In other words, she holds herself responsible for not having anyone to turn to. This means that joining HO represents the overcoming of the inability to ask for help. Like Wendy in excerpt 1, she does not hold HO responsible for her recovery, instead, she considers HO an intermediate step: First she learns to become more open towards HO members and then she also hopes she can become more open with her intimates. Thus, on the one hand, Monique justifies joining HO by constructing it as overcoming the inability to ask for help, but, on the other hand, it wards off the help-question as a dependency on HO. HO is not able to solve problems, it is her who is going to deal with, or solve her problems through participation in HO. Hence, becoming a member of HO is articulated as an important step to becoming more open or as a help-service for those who seek self-help.

In excerpt 4, in which an account is again overtly presented, the same process of invoking third parties as those who are unable to help can be observed, but here, joining HO is not treated as something urgent.

Excerpt 4 (#34)

Ria: Weg aus der Bulimie

[…]

Ich suche Betroffenen, die sich mit mir chatten oder emails schreiben wollen und mir tips geben können, Erfahrungen austauschen und auch über andere Probleme reden könnnen. Ich fände es auch schön, wenn sich hier ein paar Leute aus der Gegend [*]-Stadt finden würden, dass man sich vielleicht mal treffen kann...ich fänd es einfach mal total schön, mich mit anderen Betroffenen auszutauschen, da meine Freunde und Familie mir zwar versuchen zu helfen, aber in vielen Dingen einfach nichts nachvollziehen können und mir deshalb nicht helfen können

würd mich riesig über viele Antworten freuen,

meine Emailadresse ist: [@]

Bis hoffentlich bald!!!!!!!

Ria: Way out of bulimia

[...]

I'm looking for sufferers who want to chat or write emails with me, and give me tips, exchange experiences and who can also talk about other problems. I would also find it great if a few people from the area [*]-city could get in touch, so that we could perhaps meet up...I would simply find it really great to talk to other sufferers because although my friends and family do try to help me, there are many things they simply can't understand, and, for that reason, can't help me

would really love to get lots of answers,

my email address is: [@]

Hopefully hear from you soon!!!!!!!

Unlike the previous excerpt, Ria clearly formulates what she is looking for, namely other sufferers to communicate with online and also face-to-face. Note that this direct articulation of her wishes is *not* a help-seeking question as such, but restricts it to a request for tips, exchanges and someone to talk to about other problems, which distracts from the eating disorders as the focus of this forum. She also resists any help from HO by formulating her wishes as not that urgent (*einfach mal* and *total schön*, line 5). On the other hand, Ria invokes third parties, her friends and family, as being unable to help her. Moreover, near the end of her posting, she expresses an intense need to make contact (enthusiastically hoping for many responses [line 9], very soon with seven exclamation points [line 11]). Hence, Ria, like the other novice members in excerpts 1-3, both accounts for her seeking help, but also resists overtly asking for help. This tension is reflected in the ending of her posting in which she appears desperate for contact while not asking for help directly.

I have not yet considered how these accounts are accepted by recipients. Martine (excerpt 2) received a response, which acknowledges the account of HO as the final push of support in the recovery process: *Ich hoffe und glaube schon das du hier die Kraft finden wirst die du brauchst um stark zu sein um die Krankheit für immer zurück zu lassen* (I hope and believe that here you will find the strength you need to be strong and leave the illness behind forever). Monique in excerpt 3 also receives a similar note of acceptance of her reasoning: *ich hoffe du findest hier Kraft und Mut, um aus der ES raus zu kommen... drück dir ganz doll die Daumen...*(I hope and believe that here you will find the strength you need to be strong and leave the illness behind forever... wish you all the strength you need...). These replies do not describe the HO service as help, but as a source of strength (*Kraft*).[62] Ria's request for contact (excerpt 4) is also received positively in the sense that her respondent offers to be a good email partner: *ich bin zwar nicht aus [town in Germany] oder umgebung, aber trotzdem ein sehr angenehmer mailpartner :p* (although I am not from [town in Germany] or the region, I am a very good email partner). However, being a very good email partner (*sehr angenehmer mailpartner*) is significantly different from a problem solver, or even a help provider.

To conclude, it has become clear that novice members, on the one hand, offer accounts that suit the general accountability for seeking help ("I can't cope alone," and "no one to turn to"), while, on the other hand, they avoid asking for help directly. This indicates that HO participation requires more than accountability for seeking a help service, namely accountability for not relying on HO as a help service. Put differently, participants "orient to" an ambiguous accountability, which reflects conflicting normative requirements. Generally, the requirement for seeking help is to offer good reasons for asking for help, but in HO an additional requirement seems to be that one does not completely rely on HO as a help service. Novices "orient to" HO as offering the possibility for exchange, and recipients express in agreement with this that HO can (at the most) provide strength and courage. Displaying awareness of this by overtly accounting and resisting trouble renders a novice member forumable.

---

[62] The first response to Wendy in excerpt 1 was posted by Lucy, but was retroactively deleted by her. Therefore, it is impossible to check whether Wendy ever received a first response that "accepted" her account for joining.

7.5 Analysis: Eating disorder and knowledgeability as displays of forumability

Lamerichs (2003) identified the presentation of oneself as depressed in terms of sensitivity to the norm of offering an account for being in the forum (see above). This type of account is the most frequently used in the HO forum.[63] Self-descriptions in terms of age, type and duration of eating disorders are the standard categories used in first postings and responses. They read as formulaic expressions: "I am x and have y since z." The eating disorder is often expressed using abbreviations, such as MS (*Magersucht* = anorexia) and B (*Bulimie* = bulimia), but also UG (*Untergewicht* = underweight). These are used by the members themselves, and are not the result of corrections by moderators and can thus be understood as the members' doing being knowledgeable on eating disorders. There are various facets of self-presentations as accounts that indicate the normative requirements of participants' forumability, such as being not too old, having a recognized diagnosis, etc. These can be seen as exchanges that negotiate or make the norms, boundaries or conditions of membership in HO relevant. In fact, these cases suggest that a certain type of account is normatively acceptable for the purpose of becoming a member of HO. I will first examine more closely the fashion in which participants present themselves as eating disordered without naming a potential threat to the normative requirements of forumability. This involves the display of knowledgeability and experience regarding eating disorders.

One way to account for your presence in the forum is to display *knowledgeability* of the illness. Have a look at excerpt 5 in which Lotte formulaically ascribes herself certain categories. (ms = *Magersucht* = anorexia, UG = *Untergewicht* = underweight.)

---

[63] There is even evidence that this self presentation is normatively produced at the very beginning of the posting. This is signalled by the word *erstmal* (firstly) or *erst einmal* (firstly) in the very opening of the posting. Consider the examples:

1. *Also* ***erstmal*** *hallo, denn ich bin neu hier und möchte mich* ***ersteinmal*** *kurz beschreiben.* (#19),
2. *Hallo Leute! ich wollte mich* ***erst einmal*** *vorstellen bei euch.* (#23),
3. ***Erstmal*** *ein Hallo an ALLE;* ***Erstmal*** *muss ich sagen das ich eigentlich nicht so recht weiß was ich schreiben soll da ich zuvor noch nie in so einem Forum geschrieben habe [...]*(#29)

Excerpt 5 (#32)

Lotte: hey ihr alle
[…]ich bin [18-22] jahre alt u schon 4 jahre lang ms. vor 3 jahren war es vom gewicht
her am schlimmsten, also wirklich crass UG. […]

Lotte: hey everyone
[...]i'm [18-22] years old and have already been anorectic for 4 years. it was worse 3 years ago with the weight, I mean really severely underweight. [...]

Lotte uses abbreviations as a display of being knowledgeable about the community language of eating disorders, and thus delivers a forumable self-description.[64] She specifically notes that three years ago she was extremely underweight, using the abbreviation *UG*. This addition to the presentation of the anorectic self seems to function as a display of various stages and phases of eating disorders. In other words, it enables the novice member to convey not only knowledge of eating disorder, peer group language, but also reflexivity regarding the characteristics of eating disorders and personal long-term experience with eating disorders, which establishes her as an expert concerning eating disorders.[65] Thus, although a member enacts a novice identity (which implies being inexperienced as a HO member), a self-presentation in terms of eating disorders can, at the same time, display expertise.

Knowledgeability is also implicated in self-presentations that accomplish an identity of being a former-sufferer. It *can* be expected that people in HO who

[64] In Lamerichs' data presented above, Diana displayed knowledgeability by using medical terminology (e.g., bi-polar). However, in the US forum on depression, it appeared that participants presented themselves as depressed but competent (Lamerichs, 2003). This is clearly different from the self-presentations in HO: The display of general competence does not seem to play a role in first postings by novice members in HO.

[65] Recall HO's rule about the specification of numbers (4.2). Since HO rules are not without consequences (i.e., postings or formulations that violate them are erased by moderators), it can be assumed that participants actually make an effort to obey the regulations. However, excerpt 6 displays features that can be compared (age, type of ED and duration of ED), which was not treated as a violation of the rule. Consider also excerpt 5 for participants' inventiveness to convey equivocal information about themselves. The phrase *also wirklich crass UG* in line 2 seems to violate the rule, since it invokes the critical limit of underweight. This shows not only that moderators do not always succeed in filtering out all of the problematic terminology, but also that participants do tend to use self-descriptions with comparisons. As a result, it cannot be assumed that self-descriptions are always consistent with the rules, and that participants always obey the rules. Instead, the rules must be viewed as external norms that *may* be a resource for the participants.

have managed to recover from their eating problems will no longer be interested in participating, but this is not the case. Consider excerpt 6.

Excerpt 6 (#17)

Martine: neu hier…

[…]Kurz zu mir: Ich bin [18-22] und würde mich inzwischen fast als ehemalige bezeichnen. Allerdings traue ich dem noch nicht übern weg und habe ziemlich viel Angst. (Sowohl vor Rückfällen als auch vor einem Leben ohne Bulimie....) […]

Martine: new here...

[...]About me: I am [18-22] and would by now almost classify myself as an ex-sufferer. I don't trust that though and am quite afraid. (Not only of relapses, but also of a life without bulimia...) [...]

What is interesting about Martine's formulation is that she uses a conjunctive (*würde*) and the verb *bezeichnen*. It displays a careful consideration of her position in the various, only vaguely distinguishable, sub-categories (or diagnoses) of eating disorders. The fact that *she* would classify her self almost a former sufferer also somehow questions the validity of this categorization. There is no third party invoked to argue convincingly that she has almost recovered, and she herself is very insecure about the "recovered" state, fearing both relapses and a life without bulimia. The description in which she expresses her uncertainty about where she stands in relation to the "eating disordered" category is not related to as a problem by other forum members. Martine's self-presentation is forumable and thus she is accepted as a member.

In excerpt 7 below, the eating disorder category is treated as an identity category that you can belong to, even if you no longer practice the category-bound activities anymore. A comparison with alcoholism is evoked by the metaphorical use of *trocken*. Eating disorders are treated as something you *have*, rather than something you *do*. This implies an understanding of eating disorders as an illness with "non-practical," probably psychological aspects.

Excerpt 7 (#4)

Bertha: Neues Jahr, neues Glück?

Hallo,

eigentlich bin ich "trocken": bin [23-30], habe B*, praktiziere aber nicht mehr aktiv.

[…]

Bertha: New Year, new happiness?
Hello,
actually, I'm "dry": I'm [23-30], have bulimia, but no longer practice actively. [...]

The self-presentations in excerpts 5-7 portray the novices as knowledgeable and experienced with regard to their eating disorders. They are accepted in the community without any problems (i.e., with welcomes). Moreover, former-sufferers' postings illustrate that one can be a member not only of the forum, but also of the entire category of eating disorders, *without* practicing its typical characteristics.

In the following sections, knowledgeability continues to play a role, being a fashion in which forumability can be accomplished.

7.6 Analysis: The reciprocity of being eating disordered

In many cases, the eating disorder identity of the novice (which functions as an account) is accepted by a recipient by means of a reciprocal self-presentation. Frequently, an introduction of other HO members is only produced by one other HO member. It thus seems that one response that includes a self-presentation usually suffices, as if this one respondent is representing the entire HO forum. A characteristic of reciprocal self-presentations is that the novice sees them as an act of acceptance into the forum, which I will show with excerpt 9. Excerpt 10 demonstrates that reciprocal self-descriptions enable comparison among members.

Furthermore, the reciprocal presentation usually includes the same categories as those used by the novice: Age, the duration and the type of eating disorder. This may not be surprising because in cases in which reciprocal introduction is socially expected, it is likely that the next speaker will use the same categories to introduce her/himself as the first speaker (Schegloff, 2007). Consider excerpt 8.

Excerpt 8 (#28)
Angela: Hallo, stell mich jetzt auch mal vor...
[…]Hi, ich bin [23-30], habe seit etwas über 8 Jahren ES, angefangen mit MS, dann
B**, aber die Geschichten teilen wir ja leider hier fast alle...[…]

#Lucy
Hallo Angela!!

Willkommen erstmal!!! *freu* 

Ich erzähl mal von mir, okay? Ich bin [23-30] und hab seit etwa 14 Jahren B, abwechselnd mit MS. Hab 2 stat. Theras gemacht, beide Male waren das aber allgemeine Suchtkliniken, und hat auch net wirklich viel gebracht. Leider. [...]

Angela: Hello, will also introduce myself...
[...]Hi, I am [23-30], have had an ED for just over 8 years, began with anorexia, then bulimia, but unfortunately almost everybody here shares these stories... [...]

#Lucy
Hello Angela!!
*Firstly, welcome!!! *happy** 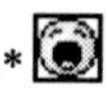
I'll tell you something about me, okay? I'm [23-30] and have had bulimia for about 14 years, alternating with anorexia. I've been to two clinics, but both times in general rehab centres, and it didn't really do much good. Unfortunately. [...]

First, Lucy offers reciprocity using the same formula and categories as Angela did (*ich bin [23-30], habe seit etwas über 8 Jahren ES, angefangen mit MS, dann B*** and *Ich bin [23-30] und hab seit etwa 14 Jahren B, abwechselnd mit MS*). Along with the personal greeting including exclamation point and the very warm welcome, the reciprocal self-presentation must be read as an act of acceptance: We share anorexia and bulimia experiences, which makes us so similar that you are as appropriate a member of HO as I am. The fact that Angela already points to the fact that HO members (indexed with *wir*) share the same stories indicates sensitivity to the relevance of similarity among members. In other words, when you present yourself in terms of the eating disorder that most members themselves have, it amplifies your chances for acceptance. Lucy's question *Ich erzähl mal von mir, okay?* (line 8) is thus (next to a topic shift away from Angela) an announcement of the realization of Angela's assumption that almost all HO members share the same stories (*Geschichten*, line 2).

Consider excerpt 9, in which the forumability is also similarly validated by the offer of a reciprocal self-presentation by a regular member. Here, it becomes clear that a reciprocal self-presentation can ward off the reading of the previous turn as a request for help. In other service provision settings (help line, doctor, therapy), a reciprocal self-presentation by the help provider is very uncommon, if not inappropriate behavior. Put differently, institutional support or help is one-directional. Despite features of accountability involved in seeking help, recipients do not treat the novice's first posting as a request for help when they offer a reciprocal self-presentation. How does the novice member deal with this?

In excerpt 9, the reciprocity is treated as an act of acceptance in the forum: Your story is like mine, so you are one of us.

Excerpt 9 (#8)

Monique: Erste Annäherung

[…]Hallo. Ich bin [18-22] Jahre (DIE Zahl darf ich wohl nennnen, oder?...:-))und hatte schon immer ein speziellles Verhältnis zu Essen. Ich kann mich nicht erinnern, dass ich nie darüber nachgedacht habe, was ich da gerade zu mir nehme, oder das es mir egal war, welches Gewicht habe und was andere von mir denken könnten. Als ich 14 war hatte ich keine gesundheitsgefährdende Magersucht, allerdings habe ich sehr darauf geachtet, was ich esse und vor allem darauf, dass ich möglichst nichts esse. Vor drei Jahren ungefähr fing dann die Bulimie an, lange Zeit nur selten, jetzt kommen die Attacken jedoch immer öfter und ich bemerke, dass ich alleine es nicht schaffe. […]

#Angela

Hallo Monique, ich bin selber [23-30] und kenne diese Art Geschichte sehr gut... bei mir hat es mit [<18] angefangen... MS und ging dann nach einer Therapie in einer Klinik recht schnell in B** über... das ist nun 8 Jahre her... immer mal der Gedanke, endlich ein "normales Leben" zu führen, aber nie die Kraft, mir meine Sucht wirklich einzugestehen und das Problem anzugehen... seit [Monat, Jahr] ist das allerdings anders...

war aber alles nicht so einfach... […]

#Monique (2)

Danke für deine Nachricht, ist schön, zu hören, dass es noch andere da draußen gibt mit dem gleichen Problem. Theoretisch weiß ich ja, dass ich mit der Krankheit kein Sonderfall bin, aber trotzdem, öffentlich wagt es kaum jemand, darüber zu sprechen. Finde es deswegen gut, dass es dieses Forum gibt. […]

Monique: First approach

[...]Hello. I am [18-22] years old (I'm allowed to mention THAT number, aren't I?...:-))and always had a special relationship to food. I can't remember a time when I didn't think about what I was eating, or didn't care what my weight was and what others might think about me. When I was 14, I didn't have anorexia to the point where it was dangerous to my health, although I was very careful about what I ate, and above all ate nothing if possible. Then about three years ago, the bulimia began, for a

long time only rarely, but the attacks are happening more and more often now, and I realize that I can't deal with it alone. [...]

#Angela
Hello Monique, I'm [23-30] myself and know this type of story very well... for me it began at [<18]... anorexia and after a stay in a clinic it turned into bulimia really quickly ... that's 8 years ago now... always the thought of finally leading a "normal life", but never the energy to really admit my addiction to myself and tackle the problem... since [month, year] that's changed, though... but nothing was very easy... [...]

#Monique (2)
Thanks for your message, it's good, to hear that there are others out there with the same problem. Theoretically, I know of course that I'm not a special case with this illness, but nevertheless, almost nobody dares to talk about it in public. Find it good, for this reason, that this forum exists. [...]

Monique displays some aspects that could jeopardize her forumability. Unlike most other HO members (both novice and regular), she does not use knowledgeability in terms of abbreviations of the eating disorders, but describes her condition as always having had a special relation to food. [66] She expresses her lack of experience and knowledge of the local rules by posing the question: *DIE Zahl darf ich wohl nennnen, oder?....:-)*, line 1. This question is followed by an ellipsis and a smiley face and works to reinforce an ambivalence or skepticism towards HO, with its elaborate Rules and Regulations. Furthermore, Monique offers trouble resistant claims, namely that the anorexia she had was not dangerous (*keine gesundheitsgefährdende Magersucht*, line 4-5), which is a way of resisting anorexia as "real" trouble, and that she managed by herself, until recently the "attacks" became more frequent. Finally, however, she literally delivers the "I can't cope alone" account (line 8), which is clearly an expression of someone seeking help. In other words, regardless of a bit of reluctance, she does display the concern of forumability. Angela, in her response, aligns herself with Monique (i.e., she writes that she knows this story very well, line 11) as a preamble to her own story.

This excerpt demonstrates that a reciprocal self-presentation is an act of acceptance of the novice member, rather than an interest in one another's problems. While Angela displayed no further interest in Monique's problems, Monique also fails to respond to Angela's personal narrative about her eating

[66] Monique earlier confided that she has read several threads from the forum (see chapter 6.4, excerpt 8), which suggests that she has read other self-presentations which included abbreviations.

problems. The reciprocity thus remains static, two separate though similar, narratives. Instead of showing interest in Angela's problems, Monique treats the reciprocal self-presentation as an act of acceptance. In line 19, she states that it is *schön* (which implies "good" but not, for instance, "very important") to hear that there are others out there (*da draußen*, line 19) with the same problem. She praises the forum for offering the opportunity to publicly speak about "the illness." In other words, the forum shows you that you are not an exception (*Sonderfall,* line 20) if you have an eating disorder. Hence, it becomes clear that one's accounting for joining the HO forum is done through self-presentations, which are mirrored by respondents, which are then seen as the creation of alliances and becoming accepted by the community. This reciprocity avoids treating the novice's self-presentation as an act of asking for help. The forum is invoked as a safe space, separate from the public in which people with eating disorders do not openly speak about their illness.

Although members usually do not openly compare their eating disorder narrative (possibly because this is forbidden in the forum rules, see footnote 65), this can be done implicitly when the novice and recipient are in very different situations or stages of their respective eating disorders. In excerpt 8, Angela and Lucy seemed to be in similar stages with regard to age and eating disorder, and the novice and regular in excerpt 9 also had a lot in common. When the eating disorder stories become rather diverse, there are some indications that this leads to comparisons among other members. Consider excerpt 10.

Excerpt 10 (#11)

Carol: meine Geschichte
[...]Ich bin [18-25] Jahre alt und schleppe die-zunächst MAgersucht-Bulimie seit knapp 2 jahren mit mir rum. [...]

#Lucy
[...]Ich bin übrigens [25-30] und leide seit gut 14 Jahren an B und MS.
In diesem Sinne... 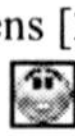
Ganz liebe Grüße
Lucy 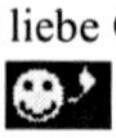
[After this no response by Carol]

Carol: my story
[...]I'm [18-25] years old and have been dragging the-initially anorexia-bulimia around with me for almost 2 years. [...]

#Lucy

[...]I'm [25-30] by the way, and have suffered from bulimia and anorexia for over 14 years.

On that note... 

Lots of love

Lucy 

In excerpt 10, again it is HO member Lucy who responds (as in excerpt 8). This time she does not *start* her contribution with a reciprocal presentation of herself, but does so at the end of the posting (after having responded to other issues raised by Carol). It is line 6, however, that renders her presentation suspicious. Lucy does not finish the sentence; rather, the interpretation is left open for Carol (and other readers) to fill in. Carol herself does not respond anymore, so it is impossible to check how she "received" line 6. It cannot be understood however, without linking it to line 5, which says (paraphrased): By the way, I am [25-30] years old, and suffer from bulimia and anorexia since over (*gut*) 14 years. Carol had earlier written that she has been dragging around her eating disorder since almost (*knapp*) 2 years. The almost 2 years stand in sharp contrast to the over 14 years. *In diesem Sinne...* (line 6) could underline Carol's hopeless prospects (that it is likely that she will also have to struggle with eating disorders for a much longer time). The emoticon suggests that Lucy is ashamed of her past of extensive eating disorders, as it shows that she is not able to get rid of them. But at the same time, it stresses her long experience.

This utterance suggests that dragging around an eating disorder for two years is not so bad compared to her 14 years. Or it may even be critical of the metaphor "dragging around" as an expression of extreme suffering, which is somewhat overdone for a person who has only been suffering from an eating disorder for almost two years. In fact, "dragging around" seems more appropriate for the one with the eating disorder that has lasted for 14 years. However, the greeting *Ganz liebe Grüße* (line 7) does not suggest that Lucy is irritated by Carol's posting at all; quite the contrary. Therefore, *In diesem Sinne...* could also just be underscoring Lucy's long-term experience with eating disorders compared to Carol, who is still relatively inexperienced. In any case, the reciprocity of self-presentations in terms of eating disorders is not necessarily only a formal procedure to offer the novice member an impression, a face of the HO members and thereby accept her/him. Although the HO rules forbid a comparison of eating disorder features, members in their descriptions do get away with it sometimes. The next section shows that having an eating disorder experience that is categorically different from those of most other HO members does not only lead to (implicit) comparison, but requires an extensive display of accountability.

7.7 Analysis: A diagnosis as minimum requirement for forumability

Presenting oneself as a member of the eating disorder category, which all of the above novice members do, is usually limited to a certain type of eating disorder such as anorexia (excerpt 5 *ms*) and bulimia, or both (excerpt 8). In the following three sections (7.7 through 7.9) I will show what happens when the novice member does not present her/himself as unconditionally eating disordered. A case in point is Lili's first posting. The eating disorder known as Binge Eating Disorder appears to cause trouble, probably because it is less well-known than anorexia and bulimia. This excerpt demonstrates that an eating disorder diagnosis is the minimum requirement for forumability.

Excerpt 11 (#25)

Lili: Neu Hier! BED?
Hallo Ihr Lieben,
weiß nun endlich was mit mir los ist. das hat irgendwie jahre gebraucht und eine gute psychologin, die mir den spiegel vorgehalten hat. nun weiß ich endlich auch, dass binge eating eine krankheit ist und mir geholfen werden kann. vorher habe ich die ganze sache gar nicht gekannt. ich dachte so lange ich das ganze essen noch bei mir behalte, bin ich doch noch nicht krank?? dann ist es doch nur frustessen und das kann ich doch ändern?? aber irgendwie kam ich nicht raus aus der ganzen sache. [...]

#25 Sara
Hallo Lili!
Willkommen hier!
Wie alt bist du denn?
Ich hatte wohl auch mal sowas in der Art wie BED. Naja, mittlerweile habe ich Bulimie. Und seitdem in etwa mache ich auch eine Therapie, ich haette mich vorher nie als "krank" oder so betrachtet, es war, wie wenn ich das mit dem kotzen irgendwie "gebraucht" habe, um zu sehen, dass ich ein Prblem habe... [...]

#25 Joe
hallo Lili,

von mir auch ein großes Herzlich Willkommen,
Also bei mir war das wohl auch bevor ich in die MS gerutscht bin auch eine art BED ich aß bis es nicht mehr geht hatte auch nie danach K*** müssen naja dementsprechend kam ich schnell ins starke ÜG und bei mir fing das dann an mit ner diät und bin mittlerweile auch knapp an der Grenze zum UG und das innerhalb kurzer zeit doch

mittlerweile ist das wie ein rausch und leider kommen immer längere Hungerphasen hinzu manchmal bis mein Kreislauf nicht mehr mitspielt. [...]
(After this no response by Lili)

Lili: New Here! BED?
Hello my dears,
know now finally what's wrong with me. somehow that's taken years and a good psychologist to hold a mirror up to me. now i also finally know that binge eating is an illness and i can be helped. i knew nothing about it before. i thought as long as i keep down all the food, i'm not ill yet?? then it's only eating out of frustration and i can change that?? but somehow i couldn't get out of the whole thing. [...]

 # Sara
Hello Lili!
Welcome here!
How old are you then?
I certainly used to have something like BED. Oh well, by now I have bulimia. And roughly since then I'm in therapy, I never would have seen myself before as "ill" or something, it was as if I had somehow "needed" the throwing up to see that I have a problem... [...]

 # Joe
hello Lili,
also a big Warm Welcome from me,
So for me it was also certainly a type of BED before i slipped into anorexia i ate till i couldn't any more also never had to throw up afterwards well accordingly moved quickly into being heavily overweight and for me that began with a diet and by now am almost on the border of being underweight and that within a short period of time but by now it's like intoxication and unfortunately there are longer and longer phases of starvation as well sometimes till my circulation doesn't go along with it anymore. [...]

In the title *Neu Hier! BED?* Lili sets the tone of her first posting: Being new in the forum with an exclamation point and BED (Binge Eating Disorder) followed by a question mark. Being a novice is frequently noted in the titles of first postings (see chapter 6). However, BED with a question mark added is quite remarkable. In line 2-3, it appears that Lili *knows* she has BED, which implies that the question mark does not mean that Lili is unsure about whether she has BED. It appears to address the fact that she *has been* unsure about whether she has BED or not. The uncertainty of the past is contrasted by a reference to the present in both lines 2 and 3 (*nun*).

Lili explains why she did not know what she had. She thought as long as she did not vomit, she was not eating disordered. In other words, she used to treat vomiting as a category-bound activity of being ill. But then, a psychologist made her realize that she belonged to another sub-category of eating disorders, of which vomiting is *not* a category-bound activity. As mentioned above, invoking a third party is a common practice in presenting good reasons for a doctor's visit. It indicates that a professional has already validated the problem, which gives Lili a legitimate reason to claim that she is sick. According to Lili, carrying the diagnosis of an eating disorder means that one can be helped, that one is doctorable. Meanwhile, eating out of frustration (*frustessen*, line 6) is mitigated to *only* eating out of frustration (*nur frustessen*), in other words, not enough to be considered an eating disorder. And as long as it is merely *frustessen*, one is expected to solve it alone. In other words, this means that once you are diagnosed with an eating disorder you do not have to cope with it by yourself, hence, you can legitimately seek help.

Recall that Lili finds belonging to the category so important that she already expressed it in the title of her posting. *endlich* und *jahre gebraucht* (line 2) in the very beginning of her posting imply that it has taken a long time before she realized what was wrong with her, and that as soon as she knew it, she composed her first posting. Now she knows it, she can finally enter the HO community. Put differently, knowing to which category Lili belongs serves as her entry ticket to the HO forum. This is neither stated on the HO website, nor speculation by the researcher, but an orientation towards the category by Lili, the member, herself. Thus, this excerpt demonstrates that presenting oneself as eating disordered counts as a legitimization for joining the HO forum. The question is whether respondents will also consider this a legitimate reason.

Sara and Joe's responses warmly welcoming Lili into the community confirm that her legitimization is sufficient. They not only welcome her, but also present their personal experiences with BED-like symptoms, which creates recognition with Lili. Simultaneously however, they confirm that BED is a contested category. Sara speaks of *sowas in der Art wie BED* (line 12) and Joe of *eine art BED* (line 20). For both of them BED-like symptoms belong to their eating disorder past, presently they are "safe" in the widely accepted categories bulimia and anorexia. Sara also thought that she did not have a problem until she started vomiting (line 13-14), which stresses that she has been as ignorant about BED as Lili used to be. In her case, she *needed* vomiting to recognize she had a problem. Thus, she treats the activity of vomiting as a means to belonging to a more clearly defined eating disorder category, namely bulimia.

Being a member of an eating disorder category has been demonstrated to be a legitimate reason for asking and receiving help, but also for forumability in the HO forum. Although the HO forum does not require a concrete eating disorder diagnosis, this thread suggests that Lili joined the forum only after she understood what her problem really was. This posting therefore displays the extreme relevance of an eating disorder category for forumability and thus membership of HO. Because categories function as an account, lack of category membership in terms of diagnostic vagueness is a problem for novice members.

7.8 Analysis: Forumability in spite of multiple psychic disorders

So far, the only identity categories that appeared in first postings were eating disorder and age. However, since co-morbidity of eating disorders with psychic disorders is quite common (e.g., O'Brian and Vincent, 2003), it is not surprising that there are novice members who also address problems other than eating disorders. In excerpt 12, it becomes clear that this is not considered a threat to HO forumability. Antonia, who recounts the various "symptoms"[67] she has, "orients to" the idea that the others may think that she is *nothing but* "symptoms." What Antonia does by writing this, is pointing out that she *is* more than just problems, but interestingly enough, she leaves implicit who she is other than a person suffering from a range of psychic disorders, i.e., she does not present any other "non-pathological" activities, hobbies, or other identity markers. Rather, the sentence displays sensitivity towards the normative requirement not to overload others with your own problems. However, co-morbidity is not articulated as problematic in HO. Consider excerpt 12 for an understanding of the accountability for having more illnesses than just eating disorders. (ES = *Essstörung* = eating disorder, SVV = *Selbstverletzendes Verhalten* = auto-mutilation.)

Excerpt 12 (#33)

Antonia: Hallo bin neu…

[…]Ich bin [18-22] Jahre alt und habe seit 8 Jahren eine ES. Das geht in Richtung Bulimie, manchmal habe ich aber auch Hungerphasen. Aber mittlerweile geht es mit der ES. Borderline ist mir auch nicht unbekannt, weil ich deswegen unter anderem eine ambulante Therapie mache. Vor Weihnachten hatte ich einen SVV-Rückfall, aber das

[67] Antonia uses the word *Symptomen* for bulimia, borderline and auto-mutilation, which is interesting since only the latter can be seen as a symptom, while borderline and bulimia are disorders, or syndromes. Through speaking of symptoms, however, Antonia is sensitive to the perceptibility of illnesses. By writing what disorders she has, she treats her problems as perceivable to others.

ist jetzt auch wieder ok. Naja, von meinen anderen Symptomen will ich gar nicht erzählen, weil ihr dann sicherlich denkt, dass ich nur aus Symptomen bestehe.
Liebe Grüße, Antonia :p

#Maggie
[...]ich denke, dass auch niemand denkt, dass du nur aus Symptomen bestehst.
Ich bin auch [18-22] und habe seit etwa zehn Jahren MS. Wenn du magst kannst du gerne noch ein bisschen von dir schreiben!!!
Liebe Grüsse Maggie

#Antonia (2)
Hallo Maggie,
danke erstmal für Deine liebe Begrüßung. Ich habe einen Waschzwang. Ich muss teilweise [*]täglich baden und ich gebe auch zwanghaft Geld aus.[...]

#Joe
Hallo Antonia,
erstmal auch von mir Herzlich willkommen hier im Forum.
[...]
Zitat:
von meinen anderen Symptomen will ich gar nicht erzählen, weil ihr dann sicherlich denkt, dass ich nur aus Symptomen bestehe.
Das denke ich auch manchmal von mir das ich nur noch aus Symptomen bestehen. Aber ich hab einen großen Respeckt das du trotz allem immernoch stark bist und den entschluß gefasst hast zu kämpfen, wie ich gelesen habe bist du auch in Thera?!Wegen der SVV?
Ich bin auch [18-22] und leide auch an ES seit einiger zeit auch mit Hungerphasen.
Glaube keiner denkt hier über einem man hat der oder die viele Symptome. Schließlich sind wir doch hier um über alles reden zu können oder?
Würd mich freuen auch von dir noch was zu erfahren.
bis denn
LG Joe

#Antonia (3)
[...]@ Joe:
Weisst Du, es ist mir nur so peinlich, dass ich so viel mit mir rumschleppe. Ich denke halt immer, dass andere dann sagen könnten, ob da noch mehr kommt und dass ich ja schon die ES habe und ob das nicht schon reichen würde. Aber ich suche mir die Symptome ja auch nicht aus. Aber mir kommen dann so komische Gedanken. Keine Ahnung wieso.[...]

#Joe (2)
huh
ich kann das gut verstehen, kenn das von mir ich schäme mich auch manchmal wieder über meine Problemchen mit freunden zu sprechen oder wenn ich mal wieder ein Tief habe und mich nur vergraben könnte wenn ich mal Depressive stimmung habe lasse ich mir das auch nicht anmerken um ja nicht wieder gesagt zu bekommen man ist der öde wieder was, und was denn jetzt ich kenn das aber manchmal ist das wichtig alles raus zu plaudern das kann wunder wirken. Ich kann das auch nur hier im Forum, denn Privat hat niemand die probleme die ich habe, was jetzt ES und so angeht.
[…]
Hoffe ich kann dir was helfen oder anregungen geben bis dann und
Liebe grüße Joe 

Antonia: Hello I'm new...
[...]I am [18-22] years old and have had an ED for 8 years. It's a bit like bulimia, but sometimes I also have phases of starvation. But recently it's been ok with the ED. Borderline is also not unknown to me, because I'm in therapy for that, amongst other things. Before Christmas I had an SIV relapse, but that's also ok again now. Oh well, I don't even want to talk about my other symptoms, because then you'll definitely think I consist only of symptoms.
Love Antonia :P

#Maggie
[...]I think that nobody thinks that you only exist out of symptoms.
I am also [18-22] and have had anorexia for about ten years. If you like, you're welcome to write a bit more about yourself!!!
Love Maggie

#Antonia (2)
Hello Maggie,
thanks first of all for your lovely greeting. I have a washing compulsion. I sometimes have to bathe [*]daily and I also spend money compulsively. [...]

#Joe
Hello Antonia,
firstly I also wish you a warm welcome to the forum.
[...]
Quote:

I don't even want to talk about my other symptoms, because then you'll definitely think I consist only of symptoms.
I also think that about myself – that I only consist of symptoms. But I have a great deal of respect that you are still strong despite everything and have made the decision to fight – I read that you are also in therapy?! Because of the SIV?
I'm also [18-22] and have also suffered from an ED for some time also with phases of starvation.
Believe nobody here thinks about whether we have this or that many symptoms. After all, we're actually here to be able to talk about everything, aren't we?
Would also be happy to learn something more about you.
till then
Love Joe

#Antonia (3)
[...]@ Joe:
You know, it's just so embarrassing that I drag so much around with me. I just always think that others could then tell me whether there is anything else to come, and that I already have the ED and whether that's not enough already. But I really don't choose the symptoms. But then I have such strange thoughts. No idea why. [...]

#Joe (2)
yoohoo,
I can understand that well, know that from myself I'm also ashamed sometimes about talking to my friends again about my little problems or when I get low again and could just bury myself when I'm in a depressed mood I don't let it show so people don't tell me I'm being bleak again, and what then I know that but sometimes it's important to let everything out that can work wonders. I can only do that here in the forum, because nobody I know has the problems I have with ED and everything.
[...]
Hope I can help you a bit or give you some ideas till then and
Love Joe 

Antonia opens her self presentation with a fairly formulaic self-presentation in terms of age and duration of her eating disorder. The subsequent lines are nuanced to the extent that she fits into several categories. *Richtung Bulimie* is nuanced with *manchmal auch Hungerphasen*. She does not *have* borderline, but she is not unfamiliar with it.[68] Moreover, the eating disorder and the auto-

[68] Note also that therapy has, in fact, taught her about borderline disorder, which resonates excerpt 11 in which a psychologist taught the patient that her problems are the illness BED. Apparently, psychological institutions are referred to in the

mutilation (*SVV*) seem to be under control now. These are trouble-resistant claims, which enable Antonia to convey signs of being able to manage by herself. Whereas the enumeration of her problems clearly depicts Antonia as a person in need of help, the manner in which she presents her problems resists this neediness. With the emoticon following her nickname in line 7 (*:p*) she seems to relativize or even ridicule herself. Lines 5 and 6 express her fear that *ihr*, that is, the other forum members, will think that she is nothing but "symptoms."

The preferred response to such a concern is delivered by Maggie in line 10. She assures her that no one will think that she are nothing but "symptoms" and closes her posting with an invitation to tell a bit more about herself, which can be read both as an invitation to tell more about things other than just symptoms, and as an invitation to talk more about her problems. At least, the fact that Maggie reciprocally introduces herself and overtly aligns with her age, works as an acceptance and reassurance. After thanking her, Antonia accepts the invitation to elaborate upon who she is, and details even more of her problems (line 17-18).

There are many other interesting aspects to observe in this interaction,[69] but I would like to focus on the accountability of having numerous problems. In line 31, Joe speaks on behalf of the whole forum in stating that no one here thinks that another person has this or that many symptoms.[70] Consider line 31-32: *Schliesslich sind wir doch hier um über alles reden zu können oder?* The possibility of talking about everything effectively means that, according to Joe, one will not be judged or laughed at in this forum, which creates a sense of security. By stressing that *hier* one can talk about everything, a boundary is set to the world outside the forum. The community is constructed as a delimitation of the out-group. In other words, Antonia's orientation toward the accountability of many illnesses is something that Joe

interaction to legitimate the use of the socially appropriate (medical/psychological) discursive devices, such as borderline and Binge Eating Disorder.

[69] In Joe's first response, the relational/interpersonal level is prioritized and signalled with *erstmal* (line 22). This stresses that before anything else, one first deals with the relation. Furthermore, Joe responds to the issue of having too many symptoms. He expresses recognition of the problem (*ich auch*, line 27), although his formulation of the problem is crucially different. Whereas Joe sometimes thinks that he is nothing but symptoms, Antonia's fear is that others think this of her. This difference is not picked up by anyone else. Joe's posting, in the first place, seems to be a gesture of recognition, according to the numerous uses of *auch* (line 29-30). He ascribes Antonia the strength and decisiveness to fight (things that she did not display in her postings).

[70] Joe's speaking in behalf of the forum both constructs the forum as a community and works to embrace Antonia as a novice member. See also chapter 6.

considers unnecessary or irrelevant in the forum.[71] In other words, the forum is used as a resource for denying the relevance of accountability for many diagnoses.

In the subsequent response, Antonia personally addresses Joe (*@Joe*, line 38) in a colloquial, personal style. Commencing with "You know" (*Weisst Du*, line 39) means that Antonia is about to confide something to Joe. This stands in contrast to the *ihr* of her first posting (line 5), in which Antonia expected that "they" would reduce her to her "symptoms." Apparently, she now feels safer and more secure in the forum. The fact that she is embarrassed about dragging around so much baggage (line 39) again exhibits Antonia's preoccupation with how others perceive her and her problems. The *ihr* from the first posting is now "replaced" by *andere* (line 40). It is unclear who these others are: Forum members other than Joe, or people outside the community? The ambiguity leaves both possibilities open. The sweet responses she receives enable Antonia, on the one hand, to not insult the HO members, implying that they would criticize her for having too many symptoms. On the other hand, it contributes to the exclusion of "others" from the forum and thus appraising the forum as such. It seems that Antonia has successfully entered the HO forum, and that, despite the number of "symptoms" she has, she is accepted and reassured that she is safe with HO. This leads to the conclusion that HO forumability is not threatened if you also have syndromes other than just eating disorders.

7.9 Analysis: Relativizing the impact of the eating disorder as a threat to forumability?

Presenting yourself as forumable by allocating yourself eating disorder categories can be problematic when you do not really want to recognize yourself as a member of these categories, including all of their inferences and features. One way to deal with this is to ascribe yourself a number of other (not illness-related) categories as well. However, this is considered problematic by respondents, since it implies that this person does not really recognize that s/he is ill. This appears to be the problem with Lotte's first steps in the HO forum, in excerpt 13. Her *first* posting is a "standard" presentation of the self using her age and eating disorder (line 1-2), followed by an extensive narrative about the course of her eating disorder (which includes trouble-resistant acts, such as in line 5: *UG aber nicht bedrohlich UG...*). Less than 30 minutes later she adds a second posting (line 10-19).

---

[71] This gesture of denying accountability does not occur this explicitly in excerpt 12. It is possibly a preliminary norm to know your diagnosis, and unproblematic if you have numerous diagnoses.

Excerpt 13 (#32)

Lotte: hey ihr alle (lines 1-2 also excerpt 5)
[...]ich bin [18-22] jahre alt u schon 4 jahre lang ms. vor 3 jahren war es vom gewicht
her am schlimmsten, also wirklich crass UG.
ich habe jedoch trotz allem niemals eine thera gemacht...
ich kann mir das auch momentan gar nicht vorstellen ..
momentan bin ich zwar auch UG aber nicht bedrohlich UG...
ich freue mich auf den austausch mit anderen betroffenen. wenn ihr fragen habt dann
fragt einfach drauf los...[...]

#Lotte (2)
vlt noch ein bißchen über meine person.
ich liebe es leute zu treffen u bin etwas durchgeknallt. ich fall meistens auf da ich eigentlich immer am lachen bin.
ich interessier mich für musik, spiel auch E -gitarre u so was alles.
meine kleidung ist meist von den beiden farben rot u schwarz dominiert ...
ich wohn noch zu hause bei meinen eltern was die essenssituation nicht immer erleichtert... 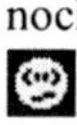
so das wars erst mal von meiner seite ...
ach u noch was wo ich grad den smiley hier seh feiern geh ich auch sehr gerne [Sektkorken Ploop!] [Breites Grinsen]

#Michelle
hey, be welcome! 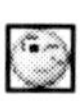
MACHST DEINEM NAMEN ALLE EHRE:
wow [contrast in nickname][72]
ausdruck deiner gefühle?
warum machste keene thera? 
ne, scherz,
aber scheinst viel energie zu haben.
so nutze sie für dich!

#Lotte (3)

---

[72] Recall that *Lotte* is a pseudonym, just like all other nicknames in the presented excerpts. The comment inside brackets is added by me (W.S.) as a circumscription of Lotte's nickname. It incorporates a striking contrast.

[…] warum ich keine thera machen will? die Es ist irgendwie ein teil von mir geworden ich kann mir gar nit vorstellen normal zu essen.. u sie bringt mein leben nicht so ins chaos das es nicht mehr lebensfähig ist...
vlt ist es naiv oder so , vlt kommt irgendwann die einsicht.. ich weiß es nicht..[…]

Lotte: hey everyone
[...]i'm [18-22] years old and have already been an anorectic for 4 years. it was worse 3 years ago with the weight, i mean really severely underweight
despite everything, i've never done any therapy...
i can't imagine that at the moment at all ..
at the moment i'm also underweight but not dangerously underweight...
i'm looking forward to talking to other sufferers. if you have any questions then just start asking...[...]

#Lotte (2)
phps a bit more about myself.
i love meeting people and i'm a bit crazy. i usually stand out because i'm actually always laughing.
i'm interested in music, also play electric guitar and that kind of thing.
my clothing is usually dominated by the two colors red n black ...
i still live at home with my parents which doesn't always make the eating situation easier... 
so that's it for now from my side ...
ah and something else as I see the smiley here I also really like to party [wine corks Ploop!] [broad grin]

#Michelle
hey, be welcome! 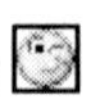
LIVE UP TO YOUR NAME:
wow [contrast in nickname]
expression of your feelings?
why don't u do any therapy? 
only joking,
but u appear to have lots of energy.
so use it for yourself!

#Lotte (3)

[...] why i don't want to do therapy? the Ed has somehow become a part of me i can't imagine eating normally at all.. and it doesn't create so much chaos in my life it's not possible to live any more...
phps it's naive or something , phps i'll understand sometime.. i don't know.. [...]

In line 6, Lotte writes that she looks forward to the exchange with other sufferers and seems to "orient to" other people's curiosity about who she is. The formulation *ich freue mich* (i'm looking forward) is noticeable, since it suggests that Lotte is introducing herself to people with the same hobby, i.e. something cheerful they have in common, and not some illness. That she is looking forward to exchange is also different from seeking help or support (see section 7.4 above). The noun *betroffenen* is ambiguous in this regard. *Betroffenen* means "people concerned" or "people involved," but also "victims." On the one hand, it is rather neutral and this allows her to avoid speaking of a group of help seekers, including Lotte herself. While, on the other hand, the victim meaning makes it clear that those people are not actors who are responsible for their own syndromes. Hence, *betroffenen* refers to those who are involuntarily caught in the same phenomenon.

The invitation that they can just shoot with their questions (*fragt einfach drauf los*, line 6-7) displays the expectation that others may have a lot of questions. Apparently, Lotte's interest is not so much that she receives answers to her questions, but that she is prepared to answer other people's questions. What kind of questions does she expect? Her second posting could reflect what she would like others to ask her. However, answering questions that have not been posed can be a delicate issue. Lotte displays uncertainty (*vlt* = *vielleicht* = maybe, line 10) about her extended self-presentation. Without giving reasons she does say that she wants to add something about herself, which implies that what she has written in the first posting about her eating problems does not concern the person she is, or is only part of who she is. What is striking about her elaborated self-presentation is the fact that the described person does not match the features generally ascribed to being ill: She loves meeting people (line 11), she is actually always laughing (line 11-12), she has various hobbies (line 13), and she really likes to party (line 18). Put differently, this additional posting is clearly trouble resistant, even directly resisting the *sick role*. This kind of energetic and positive presentation of the self is unusual in the sub-forum for novice members, which can be explained by the fact that it is not in line with the concern for forumability.

How is this seen by other HO participants? Michelle opens her contribution with a very colloquial welcome in English, possibly in adaptation to Lotte's positive and informal writing. Then she comments on Lotte's nickname[73] by hinting that the contrast (something like black-white) it embodies is a reflection of Lotte's feelings.[74] The question why Lotte does not seek out therapy (line 26) is not just an innocent question, because of the contorted face emoticon at the end of that line. Furthermore, the subsequent *ne, scherz* (line 27) makes one wonder in which sense the therapy question could have been a joke. Apparently, Michelle, on second thought, considers the question as inappropriate. Saying that something was a joke is common strategy to try to "undo" what you have said, or better, to account for what you have said if all other accounts will be considered more problematic. Retroactively, it thus considers the therapy question as inappropriate, and by the preceding *ne*, standing for *nein* (no), the question is even figuratively cancelled out, and no longer requires an answer. In line 27, the "joking" therapy question is contrasted (*aber*) with the impression that Lotte appears to have much energy. Michelle's discomfort with her own question may lie in this contrast. How can one expect a person as positive and energetic as Lotte to do therapy, purely on the basis of a nickname which suggests contrasting feelings? By the ascription of a joke to her question, Michelle has, in fact, carefully handled the situation. She ends her posting with a twist as positive as Lotte's self-presentation, not questioning the optimism, but encouraging Lotte to take advantage of her energy. Michelle's response has revealed that a highly trouble-resistant self-presentation leaves respondents with a problem, which could be described as having to deal with a lively, energetic person in an environment where one is expected to discuss problems.

Seemingly, Lotte does answer Michelle's question (line 32-35). The reason she does not want to do therapy is that the eating disorder has become a part of her, she cannot imagine eating normally and the eating disorder does not disturb her life to the extent that her life is no longer "viable" anymore. She "admits" that this may be naïve, but what Lotte types then seems to get at the central point: *vlt kommt irgendwann die einsicht...* (phps i'll understand sometime, line 35). Apparently, Lotte claims that in the case of eating disorders there should be something like an insight, an understanding, namely the recognition that you have problems or even that you are ill. Second, she renders the insight as something active that can come or go; she does not seem to be looking for it. This confession sheds new light on Lotte's positive "I am more than my eating disorder" self-presentation. Her trouble resistant self-presentation is motivated by the fact that she lacks the insight, implying she is not ready or willing to fight the eating disorder. This also explains why Lotte did not request help any earlier than in line 6-7. At the same time, it becomes clear that the only normatively relevant identities in the HO forum are

---

[73] See also footnote 72.

[74] The relevance of nicknames as self-presentations is extensively explored in chapter 5.

age and eating disorder and no other identities. These categories express an insight into the fact that eating disorders are an illness (as a opposed to a life-style, cf. *sie bringt mein leben nicht so ins chaos das es nicht mehr lebens-fähig ist...*, line 33-34), which requires treatment.

7.10 Analysis: Forumability and age

In the excerpts considered so far, it appeared that next to eating disorder categories, age is also relevant for how novice members enter the HO forum. In excerpt 11, Lili, who "forgot" to say how old she was, is immediately asked her age by Sara. In excerpt 12, it appears that age is also used in reciprocal self-presentations, since Maggie and Joe both point out that they are the same age as novice member Antonia. This means that age is used for recognition and thus acceptance.

In the first place, it thus does seem to be a normative requirement for novices to give their age. Furthermore, it appears that novice members try to justify their age if they are "too" old to have an eating disorder. Eating disorders are generally linked to adolescence, even though this is not the only susceptible age group; older, i.e., post-adolescent women and men appear to also suffer from eating disorders (Treasure et al., 2005). Nevertheless, in the HO forum, age appears to be an accountable matter. Consider excerpt 14, the opening of Veronika's first posting.

Excerpt 14 (#2)

Veronika: N'abend...

So, nun trau ich mich auch mal 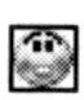
Bin nicht mehr ganz taufrisch ([35-40] Lenze) und sollte eigentlich ganz "gelassen"
mein Leben leben... Aber seit 2 Jahren beherrscht mein gestörtes Verhalten zum Essen
nun doch meinen Alltag immens. [...]

Katja
Hallo Veronika,
[...]
Herzlich willkommen hier im Forum, schön daß du dich getraut hast zu schreiben!
hier [Link], da schreiben welche die auch nicht mehr ganz taufrisch sind [Winken] .
Ich bin übrigens [23-30] und gehör dann wohl auch dazu... 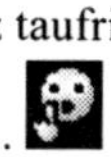
Katja [Winken]

Veronika: Evening...

So, now I'll also be brave 
I'm no longer a spring chicken ([35-40] springs old) and should really be leading my life "calmly"... But my disturbed relationship with food has governed my everyday life immensely now for 2 years.[...]

 # Katja
Hello Veronika,
[...]
A warm welcome to the forum, it's great you've been brave enough to write! here [Link], there people also write who are no longer spring chickens [waving].

I'm [23-30] by the way and also belong there myself... 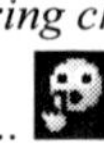
Katja [waving]

The insecurity or display of a lack of courage in line 1 is followed by the information that Veronika is not as fresh as the morning dew herself (*ganz taufrisch*) anymore. This causes a feeling of shame, as the emoticon expresses. The negation (*nicht*) constructs a contrast with those who are young, and thus implies the norm that those with eating disorders (and thus members of HO) should be young. The saying *nicht mehr ganz taufrisch* is used to refer to people of older age and the use of "springs" for "years old" is an outdated literary usage. Together, these elements articulate that Veronika thinks she is extremely old for having an eating disorder and that this is a problematic, shameful issue for her. The continuation of this sentence (*sollte eigentlich ganz "gelassen" mein Leben leben*..., line 2) displays the reason why. In Veronika's formulation, a person her age is supposed to be living a more relaxed life by now. Put differently, she "orients to" the norm that age is normative for the kinds of problems that are acceptable. People over 35 years of age should have everything under control, be cool, and take things easy, but the last two years have seen disordered eating dominating her life (line 3). The *nun doch* in line 3 suggests that, for some time, Veronika managed to control her eating problems, but not anymore. *Immens* (line 4) underlines the seriousness of this domination.

This accounting for age is taken up very cordially and reassuringly by Katja. She offers the standard welcome and a positive assessment of daring to write (cf. chapter 6). Then, she picks up on the age issue and adds a link to direct Veronika to a thread (the link has been removed and is not traceable) where presumably other *nicht mehr taufrisch*-members are gathered. It can be seen as an invitation to a (though unofficial) "sub-category" of HO, which functions as a reassurance that Veronika should not worry about having an eating disorder at her age, and that there are more like her in HO.

By adopting Veronika's formulation *taufrisch* (line 10) and by categorizing herself as one of the older ones, she is clearly aligning herself with Veronika. However, the emoticon, which implies that this information should be kept quiet, and the ellipsis in line 11 suggest that for Katja her age is also sometimes a bit problematic. In other words, Katja's reply does not eliminate the notion that being older is a problematic in this context; on the contrary, she confirms that not being young anymore *is* problematic, but says that there is another part of HO in which this norm does not matter.

7.11 Conclusion

In the overt accounts for joining HO or the displays of forumability, various strategies concerning the general accountability of seeking help can be observed, such as the preliminary expectation of having sought self-help ("I have tried to cope alone") and trouble resistant claims (not immediately consulting HO on a personal matter). However, there appear to be conflicting interests in presenting yourself as forumable. Participants do not treat the forum as a help service per se, but rather as a laudable place to exchange with others with similar problems. Overtly justifying one's participation by describing it as a step in the recovery process and resisting trouble in the sense of aiming at improving one's self-help situation seem to be the normatively required way to becoming a member of HO. In this light, not being able to cope on one's own and invoking third parties as not being able to help can possibly jeopardize one's acceptance, since these accounts for joining *suggest* reliance on HO as a help service. Since HO clearly states in its Rules and Regulations that it does not offer professional consultation and that it does not want to be a place where symptoms are discussed in great detail (these should be examined by a physician), it could be argued that overt accounts follow these guidelines.

Many novice members do not explicitly offer accounts for their taking the step to join HO, but they do offer self-presentations which display forumability. Introducing oneself through age, an eating disorder and the duration of the eating disorder is the conventional way to enter the HO forum. In many of the successful admissions to the forum the novice member receives a response in which another member first welcomes the newcomer and then delivers a reciprocal self-presentation. This is an act of acceptance, since the categorizations on the basis of which the novice member has registered are confirmed as being relevant. This means that the novice member is recognized by a HO member and thus, metaphorically, accepted in the community. The display of knowledgeability with regard to eating disorders in the self-presentation has been discovered to be a sufficient account for entering the

HO forum. Using eating disorder terminology (and abbreviations) and portraying yourself as (almost) a former sufferer invoke experience and knowledgeability and thus forumability.

Furthermore, the analyses presented in this chapter demonstrated how these normatively required categorizations can also be sources of trouble or negotiation (or exclusion, this is addressed in chapter 8). Lili (excerpt 11) only entered the forum after she "finally" understood the eating disorder that she had and thus she "oriented to" the norm of categorizing oneself with a recognized eating disorder, Antonia (excerpt 12) oriented to the norm that one is not expected to have too many illnesses, Lotte's (excerpt 13) first interaction in the forum reveals that it is accountable if you do not present yourself as a help seeker, and excerpt 14 revealed that novices orient to a norm concerning age and eating disorder. Age is an accountable matter if the participant feels s/he is too old (roughly over 30). This is an orientation to the norm that after a certain age, one is supposed to be relaxed and even-tempered, occupied with more "important" things and not struggling with issues involving eating and food. Retroactively, this renders all age presentations below this subjective age limit unproblematic, congruent with the norm. There have been no responses found, however, in which the novice member was "sanctioned" for being too old; rather, in excerpt 14, the age problem was confirmed, but the novice member was overtly accepted, reassured and invited to come join the "older" section within HO.

The example of Lili (excerpt 11), who has BED, shows that carrying a diagnosis is an account for joining HO. Diagnoses generally serve as accounts in other social contexts; put differently, having a medically unexplained illness is a source of trouble (cf. Nettleton et al., 2005). A diagnosis means being medically categorized, which facilitates social acceptance. At the same time, carrying a diagnosis means being eligible for therapy, for help. The finding that a diagnosis serves as a display of forumability in HO may not be surprising, but it is important to consider that the HO projects itself as being a low-threshold service.

The example of the novice Lotte (excerpt 13) shows how a regular member makes Lotte account for the fact that she does not do therapy. The reason Lotte offers for not seeking therapy is that her life is still livable and that she does not have "the insight" yet. The implication is that coping too well, or sarcastically put, being too "happy," diminishes the severity of the problem, which exempts Lotte from the moral obligation of seeking out therapy. Simultaneously, the account for joining the forum ("I can't cope alone") *also* goes awry. Section 7.4 revealed that accounts for joining HO describe the registration as part, or even the first step toward recovery. Countering the need for therapy thus endangers one's eligibility or acceptance in HO.

In conclusion, the eating disorder (either currently or formerly, mostly in terms of diagnosis) is the admission ticket to the forum. Despite the fact that HO projects itself as a low-threshold service for hard-to-reach people with eating problems, the interaction of novices with HO members does display certain thresholds. Presenting yourself as eating disordered is therefore crucial for novice members pursuing acceptance in HO.

Chapter 8

The main requirement of forumability: Recognition

8.1 Introduction

In the previous chapter, it was demonstrated that novice members orient to the concern of forumability by presenting themselves as eating disordered and hence, as legitimate and eligible novice members. In one excerpt (section 7.9, excerpt 13), it seems that one particular novice member did present herself as eating disordered, but also as someone possessing many non-pathological traits, features and hobbies, which depicted her as an energetic and happy person. The last part of this excerpt is repeated here as excerpt 1.

Excerpt 1 (#32)

Lotte: hey ihr alle
[…] warum ich keine thera machen will? die Es ist irgendwie ein teil von mir geworden ich kann mir gar nit vorstellen normal zu essen.. u sie bringt mein leben nicht so
ins chaos das es nicht mehr lebensfähig ist...
vlt ist es naiv oder so , vlt kommt irgendwann die einsicht.. ich weiß es nicht..[…]

Lotte: hey everyone
[…] why i don't want to do therapy? the Ed has somehow become a part of me i can't imagine eating normally at all.. and it doesn't create so much chaos in my life it's not possible to live any more…
phps it's naive or something , phps i'll understand sometime.. i don't know.. […]

In section 7.9, I argued that Lotte's "energetic" self-presentation is a form of resistance towards the recognition that she is ill. She rationalizes the respondent's question of why she is not doing therapy by writing that the eating disorder is not disturbing her life that much (line 2-3). She does recognize though that "the insight" (*die einsicht*) may come one day (line 4). The question addressed in this chapter is what the relation is between being a HO member and having this "insight," i.e., the recognition of being ill, but also needing help. Lotte's claim that her eating problems have not disturbed her life to the point where it has become unlivable constructs her as a member who is eating disordered, but not really ill.

Excerpt 1 suggests that doing therapy implies the insight that one is ill. The question of why Lotte does not do therapy thus makes this insight relevant. Apparently, HO membership can be characterized by a certain normative requirement concerning this insight. The robust nature of such requirements can be found most clearly when what is normatively expected does not occur. In chapter 7, it became clear that the eating disorder identity worked as a display of forumability, i.e., as a display of accountability for joining the forum. In the present chapter, I will look at cases in which this display of forumability is mitigated, jeopardized or absent. I thus examine what happens when novice members fail to present themselves as ill by either contending that they are normal, not ill, or pro-anorectic. I will demonstrate that it is problematic for HO as a community when novices do not portray themselves as ill. It is consequently negotiated whether the novice should be accepted or not.

Previous studies have shown that talk about being (mentally) ill involves accounting (Biddle et al., 2007; Lamerichs, 2003; Radley and Billig, 1996; D. Smith, 1978). It seems that, depending on the interest of the speaker, mental illness is constructed either as only gradually distinguishable from being normal, or, in contrast, as clearly and "factually" mentally ill. This interest is related to the relation between the interactants. As most research on this matter is based on interviews, the conversationalists can be characterized as a healthy person (the interviewer) and an ill person. Before I turn to the analysis of HO data, I will explain the potential relevance of the issues of interest and the relation between the speakers as they appear from the studies mentioned above. The data from these studies give some further indications regarding to the question of whether the allegedly ill person does therapy as part of the discussion about being ill.

8.2 Accountability of mental illness

In many cases, the development of mental illness is gradual, or, rather, the extent to which the symptoms are still normal or serious in the sense that they require medical treatment. People go through an interpretive process in which they attempt to classify their symptoms and negotiate the need for help before they actually take the step to seek help (e.g., Biddle et al., 2007) and thus socially recognize that they are ill. Similarly, others rely on lay concepts of mental illness or diagnosis before they can classify a person as mentally ill. This implies that these lay concepts are more sociocultural than individual.

At least in *talking* about mentally ill people, interactants use knowledge that they expect will be intelligible or evident to the rest. So if a person is asked why s/he did not seek help during this period of severe distress, the non-help-seeker may respond like the respondent in excerpt 2. (LB = the interviewer.)

Excerpt 2

"I didn't see it as that serious to be honest.
LB: what would make it more serious?
Um I don't know it'd just be more like being more depressed or something 'cos it isn't just like the length of how long you're depressed, it's like how depressed you get.
LB: is that why you were saying earlier it's hard to know if it's normal or not?
Yeah it's kind of like you don't know how far depressed you can get until you are that far in depressed"

Source: Biddle et al. (2007: 995).

This example shows that the severity or intensity of the symptoms (*how depressed you get* and *that far in depressed*) is a relevant criterion in deciding whether you need help or not, something that is intelligible to the interviewer, who formulates the questions in terms of degree of seriousness (*more serious*). This confirms that social actors are "sense-making agents, whose interpretative practices are informed by sets of knowledge about the world which are held in common with other people" (Wooffitt, 1992: 33). The kind of knowledge that is put to work in an interactional event depends on the "interest." In excerpt 2, the local interest is to justify why someone has not sought help.[75] It appears that a valid account would be the interrogation of the severity of the problems.

A rather different argument would be that another person is mentally ill, where the primary interest would be that the illness is constructed "as a fact" (Smith, 1978). This requires a culturally available set of assumptions about mental illness that informs both the way in which the account is put together, and the reader's interpretative practices. Smith (1978) analyzed an account delivered in a conversation (interview) between one of Smith's students (the interviewer) and Angela, who is a friend of the allegedly mentally ill woman, named K. The question which led Smith's analysis was: How is this account

[75] The interviewees were already classified as suffering from mental distress on the basis of clinical criteria, which makes it clear that the interviewer was already convinced that the interviewee was "sick." Accordingly, the interviewee was asked to explain why s/he had not sought competent help earlier.

organized to make it recognizable as an account of a young woman's decline into mental illness? So, the question is not whether K. was really mentally ill, but how a person's mental illness is discursively constructed as factual. I will briefly present some of the issues highlighted by Smith. At the heart of Angela's account was the following claim:

> My recognition that there might be something wrong was very gradual, and I was actually the last of her close friends who was openly willing to admit that she was becoming mentally ill.
>
> Source: Smith (1978: 28).

As this claim was produced at the beginning of the interview, it forms the interpretative frame through which the reader sees the abnormalities of K.'s behavior during the account. First of all, it says that besides Angela, others also considered K. mentally ill. Second, this illness is established as a fact (as opposed to a hypothesis) which is gradually "recognized" and "admitted." Third, through Angela's description of herself as a friend, the reader infers that this report of K.'s illness is not the product of malicious misreporting.[76] In the account following the claim, Angela reports abnormalities in K.'s behavior, which are frequently formulated in contrast structures. For instance:

> We could go to the beach or the pool on a hot day, and I would sort of dip in and just lie in the sun, while K. insisted that she had to swim 30 lengths.
>
> Source: Smith (1978:28-29).

In this case, the description of K.'s behavior is preceded by Angela's behavior which supplies the instructions for how to view K.'s behavior as anomalous. Similarly, such contrast structures would create the impression that what was obvious to everyone else, K. did not notice. But, in the account, K. is also presented as doing things that are motivated improperly, i.e., things that normally require contextualization, such as whispering or tiptoeing, but also insisting on swimming 30 lengths. Smith's analysis thus showed how descriptions of behavior in a certain (contrastive) structure make available inferences to whether the person can be considered "normal" or "deviant" (see also Lamerichs, 2003: 119). These inferences are connected to the culturally available knowledge of what is normal and what is not, and thus also what is an indication or symptom of mental illness.

---

[76] According to Wooffitt's (1995: 34) reading of Smith's study, the category friend also warrants authority of the account, since friends are conventionally reluctant to see negative traits, and therefore, especially as close friends, in a position to see behavioral irregularities.

The interest in designing a certain condition as possibly ill but maybe still normal, or, in contrast, clearly ill also depends on the relation between the conversationalists. Biddle et al.'s (2007) and Smith's (1978) accounts of mental illness were elicited in interviews. As scholars conduct the interviews, they also go on performing their professional tasks and thus are able to present themselves as being well enough to continue their work. Radley and Billig have addressed this aspect:

> [R]espondents with a medical diagnosis are nearly always in the position of speaking to people who are not only seen to be experts in these matters, but are also health-privileged in the interviewing relationship itself, by the very fact that the interview is taking place at all (1996: 225).

This means that when a person is classified as ill, s/he has difficulty having her/his views on other issues taken seriously. The fact that being ill is frequently seen as something amoral may also play a role. Therefore, Radley and Billig considered accounting an unavoidable part of being ill:

> Pain and associated symptoms are inescapable facts of life. What is also inescapable, however, is the necessity of appearing before others, of presenting oneself as the owner of the symptoms, the bearer of this or that illness. Giving accounts is, for both experts and lay persons, part of that business of dealing with disease and its consequences (1996: 237).

However, one cannot assume that interview settings are similar to the situation involved in writing one's first posting to an online forum. In chapter 7, I have drawn a comparison between the physician's office and the HO forum and discussed the potential differences related to the channel of the interaction (it is not possible to show bodily deficiency) and the status of the doctor as authoritative expert. During a medical consultation, the person involved was not interested in being seen as a "normal" person with opinions and views worth being seriously, but rather to present her problems as doctorable, and that s/he is justified in seeking medical attention. The interest of novice members in the HO forum to present themselves as ill (grasped with the concept of forumability) is to become accepted as a member by others with a similar condition. Hence, the interest of being taken serious does not seem to play a role in HO, at least not in the same way, as in interviews. This is connected to the relation between the interactants; there may be different interests that affect the interaction among other ill people.

Accounts of illness vis-à-vis a peer community

From Lamerichs' (2003) study, it appears that members of a peer forum on depression often portray themselves as (rather factually) depressed. They do not seem to fear the possibility that they will not be taken seriously; quite the contrary, they articulate their "different-ness" from other (normal) people as a *positive* distinction. It appears that articulating this positive feature as shared with the group works to facilitate the construction of having a depression. Hence, Lamerichs data suggest that *in a peer community* mental illness can be displayed as something positive, which does not demand the sort of accounting that interviews or other encounters with "normals" might demand. (However, note that attributing the category of "being different" to oneself is an accountable matter in itself.) The community (either the online group or all depressed people) is explicitly made relevant for this purpose. Consider the following excerpt.

Excerpt 3

Naomi:

[…] I know now, there are so many of us..I can remember the time when I accepted the fact that I just couldn't fit into a manmade mold… (and I'd tried for so long)…and you know… it felt so good..just saying it aloud. "I don't fit in this world!" Then the time came when I realized I actually liked more those who couldn't fit in with mainstream. _ I really tried…I wanted not to let anyone down…ever, and so I tried really hard and was miserable. It's hard to explain unless you already know what I'm saying… . then explanations aren't necessary.

So… . could you say that we are a group who don't fit in the

[6 lines omitted]

I went to a poetry reading once…can't even recall his name right now…but as he talked of what a poet is…how we think mosaic), feel and react…it was as though I'd come home. I'd never heard anyone say that who I was..was normal to some..that I thought the way I did because of how I was. I sat and cried while I was supposed to be taking shorthand notes. That's the reason I had gone, as a shorthand exercise for steno class. For me… . it was the most wonderful affirmation I had ever heard. I hadn't known how lacking that had been in me. I wiped tears, surprised by my emotions…and sighed deeply. I was 30 years old before I knew that I was more than just weird…

Source: Lamerichs (2003: 100).

There are a few aspects about this excerpt that I would like to mention here. The first two observations are adopted from Lamerichs (2003).[77] First being depressed is presented here as a positive attribute. Being mainstream (or "mediocrity," Lamerichs, 2003: 101) is generally not strived for, and therefore "not fitting in with mainstream" is a desired quality. Possibly negative inferences attached to being categorized as depressed are thus countered by a construction of being *positively* different from the *mainstream* and those who *fit in the manmade mold.* Second, this process is described in terms of acceptance (line 1), warding off what Naomi may have *wished* was different. Being positively different is thus presented as the realization of a gradual and difficult (*miserable*) process, which counters the intentionality or agency in becoming different and thereby renders the account more credible (cf. Widdicombe and Wooffitt, 1995). Third, two specific identity constructions are interesting with regard to the interdependency of being normal and/or depressed. Compare being *more than just weird* (line 17) and being *normal to some* (line 12). Although Naomi prefers those who do not fit in with mainstream, she does appreciate to be perceived as normal by some. This implies an understanding of normal dependent on the setting. Whereas Naomi used to think that she was weird, she now knows that to some she is normal, and she evaluates these some, implicitly including the forum community, as positively different, by stating she likes more those who do not fit into the mainstream. This means that "being normal to some" must be distinguished from "being normal to others," such as non-depressed people, or non-poets. In other words, normal is treated as a relative term depending on the out-group. The fourth observation is related to the sentence *I know now there are so many of us* (line 1). It displays alignment with the forum members (possibly the referents of *us*, line 1) as sharing the attribute of being "positively different" with her. In sum, this posting suggests a community that is defined as not "mainstream," but "more than just weird." Although the different-ness is also fashioned to construct the illness as factual, the deviance is characteristic not for her as an individual but for the entire peer community, and is not considered negatively but positively different.

It can be concluded from Lamerichs' data that community is employed to attach an extraordinary status to the mentally ill. This observation about a particular community of depressed people has more generally been made by Goffman (1986). He states that communities of social deviants[78]

---

[77] It must be noted that Lamerich's (2003) data are probably not taken from a sub-forum for novice members specifically. At least, the concern of being accepted as a novice member is not oriented to (through insecurity, self presentation, etc.).

[78] Social deviants come together in a sub-community or milieu (Goffman, 1986: 143), and are thereby distinguished from "disaffiliates" and "cultists."

> constitute a haven of self-defense and a place where the individual deviator can openly take the line that he is at least as good as anyone else. But in addition, social deviants often feel that they are not merely equal to but better than normals, and that the life they lead is better than that lived by the persons they would otherwise be. Social deviants also provide models of being for restless normals, obtaining not only sympathy but also recruits (Goffman 1986: 145).

This means that the characteristic of "being not merely equal to but better than normals" is connected to being a community. Apparently, stigma management encompasses different orientations that depend on the social context. This raises the question of accountability for (mental) illness in a community in relation to "normality." For the analysis of HO forum interactions, it must be recognized that they take place in a setting different from an interview setting or a medical visit. Therefore, the analysis of accounts of mental illness (more precisely: eating disorders) is sensitive to orientations towards the peer community.

Finally, I would like to briefly compare the excerpts 1, 2 and 3 with regard to the connection between mental illness and seeking professional help or receiving medical treatment. In excerpt 1, "not doing therapy" was treated as an accountable issue, based on the expectation that sufferers should seek professional help. In excerpt 2, the same expectation was oriented to, but there doubt about the severity of the condition was received as an acceptable account by the interviewer. In excerpt 3, the question about therapy is implicitly avoided by constructing the depression as a personal attribute that needs to be accepted rather than a condition that calls for treatment. Naomi explained that she had tried so hard (line 4-5), which could mean she has tried to become healthy or normal through therapy, but at that point it merely underlines the immutability of her condition, and not the normative requirement or moral obligation linked to being ill to undergo treatment. Hence, in excerpt 3 the community is attended to as a bastion of peers who recognize that they are different but, in fact, "better" than mainstream people and consequently freed from the expectation that they will undergo treatment. There is no suggestion of an "insight" as a precondition for therapy, since the condition is designed as a distinctly positive identity.

8.3 Goal

The following analysis examines how the acceptance of new members is negotiated in cases where novices fail to, or refuse to subscribe to an admittedly "ill" identity. In chapter 7, I spelled out how eating disorder diagnoses appear to be an orientation to forumability. Considering this, the question is what happens to the normative requirement of forumability if a novice member only half-heartedly recognizes that she is ill or does not seem to be seeking a cure. It will become clear that if being ill is not displayed unconditionally by the novice member (and s/he thus does not live up to forumability concerns), the issue is in some cases ignored and in other cases taken up and dealt with in the subsequent interaction. There are various opinions about who should be an eligible member, despite the dubious recognition of illness. Community (membership) is treated primarily as something that does not require undergoing professional treatment, but does require the acknowledgement (and thus display) of being ill.

Note that:

- Nicknames are replaced by pseudonyms, and age is replaced by age groups for the sake of anonymity.
- Text inside brackets in the excerpts is either anonymized information added by the author (W.S) or the description of an emoticon/smiley.
- The excerpt codes (#...) refer to the unique position of data in the data set.
- The typing, spelling and punctuation are original.
- The English translations of postings are added for the sake of comprehension, but the original German messages are the actual research material.

8.4 Analysis: Ill or normal?

Novice members in several first postings posed the question of whether they themselves or their eating behavior was normal or ill. The novices thus make illness as an identity relevant, but do not design themselves as eating disordered in terms of anorexia, bulimia etc. (as in the cases presented in chapter 7). Nevertheless, these novice members receive responses that are merely congruent with the responses presented in chapters 6 and 7 (i.e. they frequently receive a welcome). However, these responses are not direct responses to the "normal"-question. The novice members are accepted as novice members, but are not provided with an answer to the question of whether they are still normal or ill. Since a question generally elicits an answer, the absence of a response is noticeable (see also 6.5 on adjacency pairs). The absence of an answer is even more remarkable when the question has been posed with some emphasis and urgency. This phenomenon is demonstrated in the subsequent three excerpts. First consider excerpt 4.

Excerpt 4 (#29)

Eveline: helft mir :(
Erstmal ein Hallo an ALLE
[…]
Ich fange dann einfach mal an und würde mich total darüber freuen wenn ich ein paar Antworten bekommen würde weil ich wirklich nicht mehr weiß ob ich noch ganz normal bin.
Also ich bin [< 18] Jahre alt und habe ungefähr seit 2 Jahren Essstörungen.
[…]

Eveline: help me :(
Firstly, hello to EVERYONE
[…]
I'll just begin then, and would be really happy if I received a few answers because I really don't know any more whether I'm totally normal.
So I'm [< 18] years old and have had an eating disorder for about 2 years.
[…]

In the remainder of the posting, she repeats the question posed in line 4-5, and this time with a very strong orthographic emphasis: *das ist nicht ganz normal oder?????????????????????????????????* (that is not really normal, is it???????????????????????). Due to the repetition of the question and the orthographic stress, the question of normality is articulated as highly relevant in this first posting. However, despite its relevance, Eveline does not receive any response in which the question is answered or more generally taken up as an issue. A similar orientation to the question of normality is observable in the first contribution of Laura to the forum. Consider excerpt 5.

Excerpt 5 (#27)

Laura: bin neu
Hi Leute!

Bin zufällig aud diese Seite gekommen und ich hoffe, ich finde hier hilfe.
Ich bin erst [18-22] und habe schon so lange ich zurückdenken kann Essstörungen.
Ich habe ständig das verlangen etwas zu essen.
Am liebsten Nasche ich etwas.
Kaum habe ich etwas fertig gegessen, brauche ich gleich noch etwas.
Beim Einkaufen muss auch immer ne Extrapackung Chips oder Schokolade mitgehn.
Ist das normal?
Hoffe bald Antworten zu bekommen.

11
12 lg Laura

Laura: I'm new
Hi People!
Came across this site by accident and I hope I can find help here.
I'm just [18-22] and have had eating disorders for as long as I can remember.
I constantly have the desire to eat something.
What I most like to do is nibble at things.
I've hardly finished eating something when I need something else.
When shopping I always have to get an extra bag of chips or chocolate.
Is that normal?
Hope to get some answers soon.
love Laura

Several aspects that are noticeable about this posting were already examined in chapters 6 and 7;[79] here I will focus on the question posed in line 9. Since Laura does not say what type of eating disorder she has, her posting suggests that she has never been professionally diagnosed, nor undergone treatment.[80] Consequently, she does not know whether she is entitled to bear the label "eating disordered," which renders the question "Is this normal?" an appropriate issue of concern. The position of the question in the posting stresses its relevance, and creates the impression that this is her reason for writing to the forum in the first place. Despite her description of always having the desire to eat, she asks whether this is normal. It seems that Laura "orients to" a flexible concept of normality, in which it is possible that a constant desire for food could still be considered normal. Cultural knowledge about eating habits includes that it is "normal" to have phases or days when one has an endless appetite, especially for sweets, potato chips, etc.

On an interactional level, there are a few aspects I would like to highlight. By posing the normal-question to the forum, Laura addresses the other forum participants as being in the position to judge her condition, hence as experts.

[79] The subject line immediately stresses Laura's situational identity of being a novice member, the greeting is highly colloquial, and the opening is not the typical kind of insecurity, but a clear account for joining, namely hoping to find help. Usually, age and diagnosis are presented subsequently, which is slightly different here. Laura is only [18-22] and has eating disorders as long as she can remember.

[80] The fact that she says she has eating disorders (line 4) must not be understood as a clear diagnosis (cf. "I have bulimia"), but is the introduction to a description of her eating behavior and desires, which offers the readers an impression of her condition.

The account that she is looking for help (line 3) is a problem orientation that sustains legitimacy (i.e., forumability). In the reply to Laura's posting (not presented here) the "normal"-question, so prominent in her posting, is not answered. The reply offers a reciprocal self-presentation and a "continuer" like: "Would you like to tell a little bit more about yourself?" Hence, forumability does not seem to be critical or jeopardized in Laura's case.

A variation of dealing with the question of normality is the question of illness. An example is the question posed in line 13 of Elly's first posting, which also does not receive an answer from potential respondents.

Excerpt 6 (#19)

Elly: Was ist das?? GEFAHR?

Also erstmal hallo ,denn ich bin neu hier und möchte mich ersteinmal kurz beschreiben.

Ich bin [< 18] Jahre alt komme aus [Bundesland] und weis nicht was ich denken soll

Ich kontrolliere schon seit ca. 1 jahr mein Gewicht sehr doll. Das hat angefangen als mein Bruder aus dem Urlaub wiederkam ,er war mit einer jugendreise unterwegs und da schmeckte das essen wohl garnicht... somit hatte er dan * kilo in [zeit] abgenommen da wa ich dan sogeschockt,weil ich da nu noch * kilo leichter war.Das hat mir dan das gegeben das ich auhc nur ncoh wenig gegessen habe... mitlerweile denke ich esse ich wieder ein bisschen mehr aber seit dem [bestimmte lebensmittel nicht] mehr.Zumit esse ich wenn ich bei Freunden bin ,egal wielange garnichts.Letztens war ich [zeit] weg und in der Zeit habe ihc nichts gegessen udn kaum getrunken.Wenn ich jedoch zuhause bin esse ich schon und darunter meistens leider auchd as falsche wie Schokolade.

Einige Eltern meiner Freunde meinen ich seie "krank" und ein Freund von mir ebenso.

Was denkt ihr?

Mfg Elly

liebe elly,

herzlich willkommen im forum. ich habe die zahlen- und lebensmittelangaben aus deinem beitrag genommen, siehe unsere regeln , damit andere usern nicht zu vergleichen verleitet werden.

liebe grüße, kira

Elly: What is that?? DANGER?
So firstly hello ,because I'm new here and first of all want to describe myself a bit.
I'm [< 18] years old come from [federal state] and don't know what to think 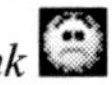
*I've been checking my weight like mad for about 1 year. That began when my brother came back from holiday ,he was traveling with a youth group and the food there tasted really bad... so he lost * kilos in [time] and I was soshocked then,because I was only * kilos lighter.That then led to me also only eating a little bit... now I think I eat a bit more but since then no more [particular food]. So I eat absolutely nothing when I'm with friends ,no matter for how long.Lately I was away for [time] and in that time I didn't eat anything and hardly drank.When I'm at home though I do eat and then unfortunately mostly the wrong things like chocolate.*
Several of my friend's parents think I'm "ill" and a friend of mine, too.
What do you think?
Best wishes Elly

dear elly
a warm welcome to the forum. i have taken out the details of numbers and food from your post, see our rules, so that other users are not tempted to make comparisons.
love, kira

Here, the novice member does not ask whether she is (still) normal, but whether the forum members think she is ill. The severity of the description of her eating behavior (line 3-11) sets up a clearly preferred affirmative answer to the question, since not eating anything when not at home is known to be highly unusual. Note that ill is typed in quotation marks (line 12), which suggests that it should not be read literally. *GEFAHR* (danger) in the title can be seen in relation to *"krank"* in line 12, which means that being ill is constructed as dangerous. *GEFAHR* in all capital letters can be read as fear, as a threat. Linking illness to danger suggests that the problem is acute and possibly requires urgent intervention in order to "rescue" this person. The invoked third parties, parents of friends and a friend, increase the legitimacy of entering the forum and posing this question (see also section 7.4).

In terms of member identities, the HO readers are constructed as experts that are able to make a diagnosis, while Elly is constructed as ignorant, which is especially evident from the subject line. Asking *Was ist das?* (subject line) suggests Elly does not know what is wrong with her, and that she needs the forum for an answer rather urgently. Despite a short welcome and a correction from a moderator at the bottom of her posting (line 17-21), Elly does not receive any replies. For whatever reason, the question of whether she is ill remains unanswered.

To conclude, some novice HO members write their first contribution to pose the question of whether they are (still) normal or ill. The position of the question in the turn and orthographic emphasis render it highly relevant. In other words, its relevance can be seen as "the reason for posting," cf. "reason for the call" (Schegloff, 1968). Hence, the other forum participants are treated as experts on this matter, and are in a position to categorize the eating behavior as either still normal or already ill. These recipients, however, do not respond to these pleading questions (i.e., responses are noticeably absent) while they do perform common actions (reciprocal self-presentation and a welcome in the case of Eveline in excerpt 4 and Elly in excerpt 6). Thus, the question of whether someone is still normal is not addressed by the recipients.[81] Searching for an explanation would be speculative, but the observation that it is not addressed or simply ignored is sufficient to recognize the significance of a case in which it *is* eventually addressed.

8.5 Analysis: "Admit that you are ill"

While in the excerpts above the question concerning normality or illness was not addressed by the recipients, in this section I take a closer look at a case in which the topic of illness is highly relevant to the ensuing interaction and eventually for the novice's membership. In this section, the novice member is indirectly rejected from the forum because she failed to recognize her illness. Consider the first posting composed by novice Sylvia.

Excerpt 7 (#31)

Sylvia: bin ich gefährdet?
hallo ihr forumaner...
also eigentlich weiß ich gar nicht genau was ich hier schreiben soll
eigentlich will ich wissen ob andere meine gedanken krankhaft finden
also ich hab meine gedanken noch nie wirklich jemanden so offengelegt was dieses
thema betrifft
weiß nicht so genau wo ich anfangen soll
also ich bin dünn eigentlich habe ich auch untergewicht
ich wiege mich [*] mal täglich und ich muss immer mein gewicht genau kennen wenn
es morgens mehr ist dann krieg ich immer angst das ich zunehmen könnte

---

[81] Furthermore, it must be noted that, in comparison to the replies to other first postings, the replies are short.

ich esse eigentlich normal aber ich finde fleisch manchmal richtig wiederwärtig auch kann ich sachen nicht essen die über dem mindesthaltbarkeitsdatum sind
ich möchte eigentlich noch dünner sein aber ich habe noch nie bewusst abgenommen und auch noch nie bewusst weniger gegessen
dennoch wünsche ich mir manchmal irgendeine krankheit zu haben (zB magen darm grippe) wo man natürlich und somit von außen gesehen "echt" abnimmt wisst ihr was ich meine?
also so das ich niemanden erklären muss warum ich jetzt abgenommen habe
manchmal hab ich den drang mich zu schneiden nicht doll meistens [Beschreibung Selbstverletz. Verhalten]
ich finde mich persönlich zu fett ich kann manchmal sehr lange im spiegel mich an-gucken und denk dann "ie wie fett bist du wie fett sind deine oberarme" aber meine oberarme sind wirklich fett also so richtig eklig
naja
ich war mal eine zeit lang blutspenden aber ich wurde gesperrt weil ich angeblich zu dünn sei
mein gewicht ist aber eigentlich normal
und wie gesagt ich hab noch nie bewusst abgenommen und ich esse auch eigentlich gern nur halt die ekligen sachen nicht so gern
ist das jetzt krank? ich mein irgendwie ist es schon krank...aber ist es SO krank?
ist es krank zu denken zu hoffen das man irgendwie doch noch dünner wird????
ich dank euch schon mal
[Liebe Sylvia. Bitte keine Zahlenangaben zu deinem Gewicht oder was damit zu tun hat und keine Beschreibungen wie du dich Verletzt. Lies dir doch nochmal die Regeln durch. Liebe Grüße Marcia]

Sylvia: am I at risk?
hello you forumers...

so i don't actually know what i should write here exactly
actually i want to know whether others find my thoughts abnormal
so i've never really revealed my thoughts to anyone on this subject
don't really know where to begin
so i'm thin actually i'm also underweight
i weigh myself [*] times daily and i always have to know exactly what my weight is if it's more in the mornings i get frightened i could put on weight
i actually eat normally but i sometimes find meat really repulsive and i also can't eat things that have gone beyond the best before date
i actually want to be thinner but i've never lost weight intentionally and also never eaten less intentionally

nonetheless i sometimes wish i could get some kind of illness (eg stomach flu) where it's possible to naturally and from the outside "genuinely" lose weight do you know what i mean?
so in such a way i don't have to explain to anyone why i've now lost weight
sometimes i have the compulsion to cut myself not badly usually [description of self-harming behavior]
i personally think i'm too fat i can sometimes look at myself in the mirror for a long time and then think "ugh how fat you are how fat your upper arms are" but my upper arms really are fat – really disgusting
oh well
i used to donate blood for a while but i was banned because i'm apparently too thin but my weight is actually normal
and as i said i've never lost weight intentionally and i also actually like eating just not the disgusting things as much
now is that ill? i mean somehow it is actually ill…but is it REALLY ill?
is it ill to think to hope that one somehow will eventually get thinner?
thanks in advance
[Dear Sylvia. Please don't give any figures for your weight or anything to do with it and no descriptions of how you harm yourself. Read through the rules again. Love Marcia]

There are many aspects in this posting that are related to the analyses found in chapters 6 and 7, such as the subject line invoking a sense of danger as a relevant category, the greeting as making the location of the interaction relevant but, at the same time, creating distance between herself and the forum members, and the production of intimacy by confiding something that she has never shared with anyone before. Moreover, Sylvia reveals insecurity in the opening line (line 3) as most novices do (chapter 6). Subsequently, however, she does *not* introduce herself in terms of age, eating disorder and duration of eating disorder. This difference appears to be explained by the fact that she does not know whether she has an eating disorder. More precisely, she is not sure whether she is really ill or not.

The question of illness appears to refer to an array of dimensions. In line 4, the question concerns the "illness/ abnormality of thoughts" while Sylvia characterizes her eating behavior as normal (line 11 and 27). In line 7, she states that she is underweight, but in line 24 she claims that her weight is actually normal. This seems contradictory. Apparently, according to medical standards, she is underweight, but in her own eyes her weight is normal. However, the blood donor center rejected her because she was allegedly (*angeblich*) too thin. Although *angeblich* indicates that Sylvia is skeptical about the ground for the rejection, by admitting the blood donor center's assessment of her body weight as too low she offers the HO participants an indication that she is factually underweight. On the other hand, she personally *finds* herself too fat (line 21) and in response, she seeks to lose more weight. In sum, this posting reveals a differentiation between the medical (and thus socially authoritative) perspective on Sylvia's condition and her personal perspective. The personal perspective (not being that ill, or not ill at all) is supported by the fact that she does not like meat, would not eat products which have reached their expiration dates (line 11-12) or that are disgusting (line 29) and has never consciously dieted (13-14). The socially authoritative perspective is represented by a medical vocabulary (*UG*) or by professionals (the blood donor center employees). Thus, categories are employed to set up two versions of Sylvia's condition. In other words, Sylvia herself offers the resources for others to actually think she is ill.

By asking whether this is really ill, she offers others the option to disagree with her personal perspective. In fact, she even admits that somehow her condition is ill (line 30) followed by: *aber ist es SO krank?* (line 30). This displays a gradual understanding of illness, articulating the relevance of the degree of illness, rather than illness as a fixed, demarcated category. The question is very important and, taking into account the position within the posting and the orthographic stress (question marks), it enhances the interest in understanding the issue of being ill or *that* ill. Obviously, one may wonder what Sylvia wants from the HO forum, since it is unlikely that other members would be able to calm her down by saying that she is not sick and could continue to lose weight and mutilate herself. This raises the question of how HO members deal with a novice that presents herself as ill (related to medical standards and practices socially known as not normal, such as self-harm), but at the same time as not willing to view herself as ill. In section 8.4, we saw cases where asking the question about being ill or normal went unaddressed by the respondents. In this case, it *is* addressed. See excerpt 8.

Excerpt 8 (#31) Continuation of excerpt 7.

Jennifer (1)

Hallo,
ich habe Deinen Beitrag gelesen und dachte mir ich schreib Dir mal.
Ich habe mich in einigen Dingen was Du geschrieben hast wieder gefunden.....
Jeden morgen auf die Waage stellen das mache ich auch.
Dünner sein wollen...ist wohl auch wieder mein Ziel.
Ob das krankhaft ist...?
In gewisser weise denke ich das sowas nicht normal ist, momentan ist mir das aber relativ egal.
Seit wann hast du diese Gedanken? [...]

Sylvia (2)
hmmm keine ahnung
irgendwie schon lange...also so einige jahre bestimmt
ich weiß nicht warum das so ist....aber mir eigentlich ist es mir auch egal so wie du geschrieben hast
mich hat nur interessiert ob das schon ein bissl crazy ist was ich mir da denke...
ehrlich gesagt würde ich mich sogar freuen wenn mir jemand sagt das er findet ich sei zu dünn
aber das mit dem ritzen ist auch komisch weil ich mach das einfach so ohne grund manchmal hab ich
einfach bock darauf...
[…]

Sylvia (3)
@Marcia: entschuldigung, ich hatte zwar die regeln gelesen aber ich hab dann irgendwie nich so
genau drauf geachtet..also ich habs schon versucht aber das muss ich dann wohl überlesen haben

Jennifer (1)
Hello,
I read your post and thought I'd write to you.
I saw myself in many of the things you wrote about.....
Standing on the scales every morning – I do that too.
Wanting to be thinner…is definitely also my goal.
Whether that's abnormal…?
In a kind of way I think that things like this aren't normal, but at the moment I don't really care.
How long have you had these thoughts? […]

Sylvia (2)
hmmm no idea
somehow quite a long time...so definitely several years
i don't know why it's like that….but for me actually i also don't care just like you have written
i was just interested whether it's a bit crazy what i think…
to be honest i'd even be happy if somebody told me that they think i'm too thin
but the cutting is also strange because i do that simply without a reason sometimes i simply fancy it…
[…]

Syliva (3)
@Marcia: sorry, i did read the rules but i then somehow didn't stick to them exactly..i mean i did try but i must have overlooked that

First, one notices that Sylvia is not being offered a welcome, which suggests that she is neither (yet) being treated as a HO novice member, nor does she receive any reassuring remarks in reaction to the displayed insecurity together with the announcement of confiding something personal (line 4-6) (see 6.5 about insecurity and being welcomed). By contrast, Jennifer formulates her reply in a slightly disinterested manner (*dachte mir ich schreib Dir mal...*, line 33) and does not treat Sylvia's first posting as an urgent request (*mal* implies no urgency). Jennifer at least mitigates the relevance of the question of illness (line 38-39) by expressing that it is not relevant for her at this moment. This can be read as a dispreferred (and face-threatening) response, because Jennifer is an experienced HO member who is not posting in the sub-forum for novices to discuss her own problems, but to deal with an "application" by a novice. Hence, it implies that Sylvia's question is not quite the appropriate question to ask. Sylvia, in turn, reformulates her question in line 47, but now more colloquially (*ein bissl crazy* vs. *krank* and *krankhaft* in the first posting) and in a mitigated form (*nur*, *schon, bissl)*, which downplays its seriousness (the same for the issue of self-mutilation in line 50-52 for which she uses more colloquial forms: *ritzen*, *bock*).

Hence, Jennifer's rejection of the question of illness constructs a problematic position for Sylvia, which she responds to by using a mitigated reformulation of her question. It is notable, however, that although she agrees with the question's irrelevance (line 45-46), she perseveres, poses it again, and continues to return to it in her other contributions (excerpt 10 and 11). In the subsequent contribution by Jennifer (excerpt 9), she does provide an answer to the illness-question indirectly.

Excerpt 9 (#31) Continuation of excerpt 8.

Jennifer (2)

[…] Warum man sich wünscht dünner zu sein?....Vieleicht weil man entlich was kann, was andere "normalesser" nicht können.
Oder ein Beweis: Das man damit sagen will "Hallo hier ist auch noch wer und bin auch was besonderes, was einmaliges?"
Hast Du schon mal eine Thera gemacht oder es zu mindestens in betracht gezogen?
Weil ich denke was wir machen ist kein normales Verhalten...Egal wie schlimm es ist...Es ist ja schlimm genug das man sollche Gedanken hat und wenn man sie Täglich hat sich auf nichts anderes Konzetrieren kann, sondern nur auf z.B die Waage, abnehemen, wie esse ich, was esse ich, vieviel esse ich u.so.w auch SVV ist nicht gerade normal und wird denke ich auch eine Usache haben - denn ohne einen Grund macht man sowas nicht, auch wenn einen der Grund nicht gleich einfällt/auffällt. […]

Jennifer (2)

[…]

Why does one wish to be thinner?....Perhaps because one is finally able to do something which other "normal eaters" can't do.

Or it's a statement: We want to say "Hello here is somebody and I'm also something special, something unique?"

Have you already done any therapy or at least considered it?

Because I think what we do is not normal behavior...It doesn't matter how bad it is...It's bad enough that we have such thoughts and if we have them daily we can't concentrate on anything else except eg the scales, losing weight, how I eat, what I eat, how much I eat etc. SIV also isn't exactly normal and I think will also have a cause – because we don't do something like that without a reason, even if the reason doesn't immediately strike us/stand out.

[…]

The question of whether Sylvia does therapy is accounted for with the claim that what "we" think is not normal behavior irrespective of the degree (*Egal wie schlimm es ist…*, line 59). She explains that this is true for both eating disorders and self-mutilation (line 59-64). This means that Jennifer denies that the degree of illness (cf. *SO krank*) is relevant, but that one thing is clear: What "we" do is not normal, thus "we" are ready for therapy. She also attends to the "culturally available knowledge" that self-injury is not quite normal (*nicht gerade normal*, line 62).

In terms of situational identities, several aspects can be observed in Jennifer's posting. First, Jennifer acts as an expert on the topic of eating disorders by explaining the desire to become thinner (line 54-57). In fact, this type of reflection on and understanding of eating disorders sounds like expert or therapy discourse by the use of rhetorical format (posing a question and subsequently answering it) and the choice of the 3rd person singular pronoun that constructs this to be a general characteristic of eating disorders as opposed to a personal experience or opinion. Thus, Jennifer treats Sylvia as a person in need of an explanation and as someone who is ignorant regarding the essence of eating disorders. At the same time, the *wir* in line 59 unites Jennifer and Sylvia (or the whole HO community, or all people with eating disorders) as having something in common which is not normal. Thereby she ascribes not only to Sylvia not being normal, but also to herself (or all HO participants, or all sufferers of eating disorders), which mitigates the face-threat of the ascription. In other words, Jennifer has shifted the focus of the issue of illness to "not normal behavior" irrespective of its degree and its implication, namely the need for therapy. At the same time, she has constructed Sylvia as sharing this "not normal" feature with the other forum members, which can be read as (temporary) inclusion of Sylvia in HO. Subsequently, Sylvia indirectly refuses inclusion in Jennifer's *wir*. Consider excerpt 10.

Excerpt 10 (#31) Continuation of excerpt 9.

Sylvia (4)
64 naja es dreht sich bei mir nich den ganden tag um essen und gewicht und so was
65 [...]
66 aber ich mein warum soll ich ne thera machen? was soll ich da? ich mein ok ich
67 scheind mich ab und an mal ein bissl..aber das hat noch keiner mit gekriegt
68 und was soll ich denn da erzählen? das ichn bissl bescheuert im kopf bin?
69 und ich denke es geht viele vielen in diesem forum schlechter als mir..und ich mein
70 ich kotze nich ich ess nicht nichts und auch so?
71 also ich mein so krank bin ich doch gar nicht oder?
72 ich mein normal ist das auch nicht aber auch nich unnormal odeR
73 wie alt bist du eigentlich?
74 ich bin jetzt schon über [18-22]...also schon kannste streichen

Sylvia (4)
well my whole day doesn't revolve around food and weight and that kind of thing
[...]
but i think why should i do therapy? what would i do there? i mean ok i cut myself
every now and again a little bit..but nobody has noticed that
and what would i tell them? that i'm a bit stupid in the head?
and i think there are many in this forum who are in a worse state than me..and i mean
i don't throw up i don't eat nothing and all that?
so i mean i'm not actually that ill, am i?

i mean it's not normal either but also not abnormal, is it?
how old are you actually?
i'm already over [18-22]... so you can cross out already

Sylvia denies that she is always thinking about food and her weight (line 64), but paradoxically emphasizes how it does occupy much of her mind. Since she does not vomit and does eat, she concludes that she is not that ill (line 71). In other words, by stressing that she does not do what she understands to be (category-bound) activities connected with eating disorders, she has an argument for claiming that she is not *that* ill, and thus implicitly denies that she really has the desire to become a HO member. Furthermore, in line 66 Sylvia treats the option of therapy for herself as something ridiculous, referring to the moral connotation of malingering, which is acted out by denying illness. Only being a *bissl bescheuert im kopf* (line 68) is not enough to legitimately seek medical treatment. Moreover, with line 72 she reintroduces a scale of illness, which she explains further by asserting that it is neither normal nor abnormal (*unnormal*). Put differently, Sylvia constructs ill as a gradual category and herself as, though not normal, not abnormal either, but she also asks for affirmation of this position (*oder?* in lines 71 and 72). Interestingly, she does not yet give reasons why the self-mutilation would not be that ill (but she does that later in the interaction, line 94).[82] The discussion continues with a posting by Joe (excerpt 11), who adds another perspective on the issue of illness and normality, namely health.

Excerpt 11 (#31) Continuation of excerpt 10.
Joe (1)
75 [...] Denke schon das es nocht genz gesund ist was du dir da überlegst und wünschst,
76 denn das kenn ich nur zu gut denn bei mir ist momentan auch der satndpunkt immer
77 mehr abnehmen doch ich weiß das ich meinen Körper nichts gutes tue aber auch
78 gleichzeitig mich wohl fühle für jeden kilo weniger 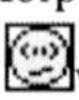verrückt.
79 Ich denke ich kann dich gut verstehen, man findet sich immer zu dick ich bin zwar ein
80 mann habe aber die gleichen probleme was figur angeht wie ihr 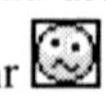
81 Ich mein ich war stark ÜG als ich anfing ne Diät zu machen und naja bin jetzt schon
82 an der grenze zum UG angekommen doch ich kann es nicht stoppen finde mich auch
83 noch richtig zu fett und da stört es mich kaum das meine klamotten alle nicht mehr
84 passen, zu groß.

[82] Note also that the identity category of age, which was not present in the beginning of the interaction, is now introduced by Sylvia (line 73-74) and is thus still oriented to, see section 7.10.

Also denke auch das eine thera in deinem falle (mich an die nase fasse) auch in frage kommt aber ich denke man muss auch 100% wollen und schaffen. Mein standpunkt ist auch wie deiner, was soll ich denn da noch fühle ich mich wohl, denke auch das mich so wie fit ich bin auch kein Arzt ernst nehmen wird, schon weil ich ein mann bin, [...]

Joe (1)
[...] I do think that it's not completely healthy what you're thinking and wishing for, because I know that only too well because for me at the moment the attitude is also to always lose more weight but I know that I'm not doing my body any good but also at the same time I feel good about every kilo lost insane.
I think I can understand you well, we always find ourselves too fat I might be a man but I have the same problems with my figure as you
I mean I was heavily overweight when I began to diet and well am now already arrived at the border of being underweight but I can't stop it also find myself much too fat and it doesn't bother me that my clothes don't fit anymore, too big.
So also think that therapy in your case (look who's talking) is a consideration but I think one has to want it and work for it 100%. My attitude is also like yours, what would I do there I still feel ok, think also that no doctor would take me seriously as fit as I am, just because I'm a man,
[...]

Joe considers Sylvia's wishes and thoughts (which are the same as his own) as not really that healthy (line 75), which he links to the body (line 77). The desire to become thinner or the idea that one is fat despite being underweight is not categorized as either ill or normal, but as not very healthy for the body. Still, he considers Sylvia (as well as himself) as a legitimate candidate for therapy (line 84-85), which can only work, however, when you are 100% motivated. Consequently, he claims that as long as you feel well a physician would not take you serious. In other words, legitimacy for therapy is linked to feeling well or not, and not to "objective" symptoms.[83] Retroactively, this functions as an account for not engaging in therapy. At the same time it

[83] Moreover, Joe also refers to his gender as accountable with regard to eating disorders. Joe is the only HO member that orients to gender in the interactional data besides through nicknames. Apparently, gender is only explicitly occasioned in the case of a male appearing in a predominantly female setting. Despite the fact that eating disorders are frequently explained by a gender specific understanding of individuals and society, femaleness or femininity do not appear as a topic in the forum for novice members (and hardly ever in any of the other sub-forums). However, gender *is* constructed through nicknames, see chapter 5.

shows that in HO, you do not have to feel very bad in order to be forumable. Hence, HO is a space for people that still feel well (*noch fühle ich mich wohl*, line 86), whereas, according to Joe, this is not justifiable when seeking help in the medical sphere. Forumability and doctorability can therefore not be equated.

Excerpt 12 (#31) Continuation of excerpt 11.

Sylvia (5)
88 […] hatte irgendwie auch heut wieder voll den drang nach SVV.[*]..aber ich habs mir
89 verkniffen
90 hmm aber eigentlich ist es doch nicht schlimm wenn ich jetzt ein bissl abnehme oder?
91 ok das ist wahnsinn ich weiß das auch selbst aber was macht das denn schon aus?
92 so bis dahin....
93 findest du wirklich das das krank ist?
94 ich mein ich esse doch...und wegen dem bissl schneiden ist doch noch keiner gestor-
95 ben
96 
97 […]
98 [Der Beitrag wurde nachträglich verändert von: Marcia]

Sylvia (5)
[…] somehow had a really strong urge again today for SIV.[*]..but i suppressed it
hmm but it's actually not bad if i lose a bit of weight now, is it?
ok that's madness i know that myself but what difference does it make?
so till then....
do you really think that that's ill?
i mean i do eat...and nobody's died because of a little bit of cutting
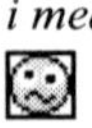
[…]
[The post was subsequently changed by: Marcia]

In Sylvia's next reply, she does not openly agree with Joe's answer and instead depicts contradictory and confusing issues. First, she returns to the issue of self-mutilation, which she describes as an urge or impulse, which she has suppressed (*verkniffen*, line 88-89), whereas later on she downgrades her self-mutilation to something not very damaging since it is not fatal (line 94). Her "personal" perspective on losing weight as not that ill is followed by the opposite (*wahnsinn*) and, despite the fact that she knows it, she contends that it does not matter (line 91). After a closing remark, she asks whether Joe really thinks "that" is ill. The emoticon at the bottom of her posting displays a twisted, blue face, graphically expressing the twists and contradictions that have also characterized her writing.

Significantly, both Sylvia's first and fifth postings (excerpts 7 and 12) are sanctioned by moderator Marcia. In the first posting, Marcia kindly (see the greeting) explains her interventions and advises Sylvia to read the rules once again. In this way, Marcia treats Sylvia as an ignorant novice member. Sylvia in line 56-59 apologizes and explains her "mistakes" by claiming she overlooked them. Marcia's second intervention is located by the asterisk in line 88 and the authorship of the intervention is added at the bottom (line 97). This intervention is not accompanied by an explanation. It cannot be traced what Sylvia originally typed but it is clear that Marcia has checked this thread (although some expressions are not censored, such as *ritzen* in line 50 and *bissl schneiden* in line 66-67). Marcia's interventions can be characterized as executions of a certain power. The original posting of the HO member is literally "broken into." Also salient is the fact that this intervention is signed by the moderator (this is not necessarily the case). This renders the activity of intervention an observable activity between identifiable members of distinct statuses. In this thread, however, the moderator decides to not only intervene unless it is absolutely necessary (which is her job), but to contribute a posting herself. If Marcia had not intervened earlier, her posting could be read as just any other member's contribution, since moderators are also HO members, and can also participate in discussions when they are not "on duty."[84] But after having already intervened in this thread, Marcia's contribution (line excerpt 13) must be read as a contribution with extra weight and authority.

Excerpt 13 (#31) Continuation of excerpt 12.

Marcia (2)

97 Hallo Sylvia,

98

99 also was willst du denn von den Usern hier im Forum hören?

100 Ich denke, dass du dich hier in diesem Forum registriert hast und dich aktiv beteiligst

101 zeigt doch, dass du selbst weißt, das dein Verhalten eben nicht normal ist.

102 Klar ist es nicht das Problem wenn jemand kein Fleisch isst oder besimmte Lebens-

103 mittel nicht mag.

104 Aber, sich ständige Gedanken ums Essen zu machen, andauernd abnehmen wollen

[84] Although moderators post "as members," they are still recognizable as moderators, since their nicknames, which appear with their contributions, are labeled "moderator."

und sich selbst zu verletzten ist in höchsten Grade nicht normal.
Ich denke es geht hier auch nicht darum was "normal" ist und was nicht.
Aber es tut dir und deinm Körper nicht gut.
Diese ganzen Dinge die du beschreibst: andauerndes Wiegen, Wunsch nach einer Krankheit zum Abnehmen, Selbsthass, deutet alles darauf hin dass du Probleme hast.
Gesteh sie dir ein und spiel sie nicht herunter.
Ich denke deine Frage ob du krank bist oder nicht kannst du dir auch selbst beantworten.

Liebe Grüße Marcia […]

Marcia (2)
Hello Sylvia,
so what do you want to hear from the users here in the forum?
I think the fact you have registered here in the forum and actively take part shows you know yourself that your behavior is not actually normal.
It's obviously not a problem if somebody doesn't eat meat or doesn't like particular types of food.
But thinking about food all the time, continuously wanting to lose weight and harming yourself is not normal to the highest degree.
I also think this is not about what is "normal" and what not.
But it's not doing you and your body any good.
All the things you describe: constant weighing, wish for an illness to lose weight, self-hate, all point to the fact that you have problems.
Admit them to yourself and don't play them down.
I think you can also answer your question whether you are ill or not yourself.
Love Marcia
[...]

In line 99, Marcia does not write "what do you want to hear from us?" but "what do you want to hear from the users here in the forum," thus not directly establishing herself as one of these users, but as someone speaking on their behalf. The question is a display of irritation, which can be explained by the fact that despite various answers, Sylvia recycled her question "is this ill?" time and time again. Now Marcia provides the definitive response quite firmly. She differentiates between unproblematic things and other things that are *in höchsten Grade nicht normal* (line 105), which, in this formulation, is not a matter of opinion, but fact. Despite this clarity, Sylvia denies the relevance of the issue of what is normal and what is not, and the point that this behavior is damaging to you and your body (note that "you" and "body" are treated as separate entities here). In other words, it is not a discussion about principles or viewpoints, but about bodily, "real" and personal mischief. She then provides a summary of Sylvia's problems and commands her to admit them to herself and not to downplay them (the use of an imperative in line 110 constructs Marcia as a member entitled to tell a novice what to do). Moreover, Marcia asserts that Sylvia, in fact, knows that she is ill twice (line 100-101 and 111). Line 111 is interesting as it is typed as the ending of the posting. Thereby it is an alternative formulation of the question "so what do you want to hear from the users here in the forum?" Both formulations underscore the inappropriateness of Sylvia's (repeated) question of whether she is that ill. The first formulation referring to Sylvia's problem reveals something else. In line 100-101, Marcia equates active participation in HO with a display of the recognition that one's behavior is not normal. This means that Marcia, a HO member with authority, treats, or even defines, participation in HO as an epistemologically performative act. Writing here in this forum is a display of admitting that you are ill.

To conclude, this thread reveals that becoming accepted as a member of HO requires compliance with or, better yet, requires the display of a certain premise. Since being an active member of HO is defined as recognizing that you are ill, a member is required to admit that s/he is ill. Implicitly a comparison with therapy is offered in the course of the analyzed thread. HO members' problems are discussed as "bad enough" to legitimately warrant the seeking out of help in terms of therapy. However, novice member Sylvia denies that her condition is serious enough to warrant for therapy. Another member, Joe, differentiates between the seriousness of the illness and the motivation to engage in therapy. He believes his condition warrants therapy, although he has not started one yet, because he still feels "too well." In other words, it is possible to admit that you are ill, without actually acting upon it by engaging in therapy.

This implies two things. On the one hand, in HO one can reflect on one's ill condition as long as it is articulated as ill, possibly also as a step toward seeking therapy. On the other hand, if a novice member does not admit that s/he is ill during her/his initiation, recipients will softly or more harshly (apparently depending on the status of the member) point out the requirement to the novice. In this case, the novice member never returns to HO again (at least not under the nickname Sylvia). Hence, in the HO forum the "community" is not articulated in terms of a positive group identity ("better than normal") as it was in excerpt 2, but it is used to settle issues of forumability which are linked to the recognition of the novice's ill condition. HO is constructed as a community that serves as a kind of intermediate step towards therapy. However, not everyone is welcome. Forumability requires the recognition of being ill, either clear through a diagnosis (chapter 7) or at least with the "insight" that one's eating behavior is not normal, is unhealthy or ill.

8.6 Analysis: A pro-ana identity in the HO forum

This section proposes to explore the role of community in the first posting of an unusual novice member (in contrast to the other 26 threads), a pro-anorectic member. Here again, the question of being ill is the novice's concern, and the community's task to deal with. In this case, the danger to forumability is similar to the one presented in section 8.5 (failing to recognize that one is ill), but has a significantly different orientation, namely the discourse of pro-anorexia. The thread is roughly structured in three dialogues, between Doreen and Paula, Doreen and Food and Doreen and Eleanor:

- Doreen (first posting) – Paula (1) – Doreen (2) – Paula (2) – Doreen (3)
- Doreen (first posting) – Food (1) – Doreen (3) – Food (2)
- Doreen (first posting) – Eleanor – Doreen (3)

Doreen's first posting addresses the whole forum, while her third posting is a response to the three recipients. Furthermore, Food and Eleanor also implicitly respond to Paula's attitude towards pro-ana (*Wahnsinn...*, line 62). I will first highlight some features of Doreen's posting and subsequently sketch how the three recipients respond to it. (FA = *Fressattacke* = binge.)

Excerpt 14 (#A22)

Doreen: ziemlich unsicher

Hallo mal an alle! ich bin mir nicht wirklich sicher ob ich hier richtig bin, mir hat ne freundin den Rat gegeben mal hier zu schreiben, es is die einzige die mich je hätte zu sowas bringen können!
Gut um es auf den Punkt zu bringen, ich bin jetzt seit einem jahr ["magersuchtsverherrlichend"], aber ich bin mir nicht sicher ob das richtig ist, und ob ich wirklich krank bin, oder nur krank sein will, das weiß ich einfach nicht, ich persönlich seh es einfach nicht ein, wenn jemand sagt, dass ich krank bin oder dass ich ein problem hab!!

Angefangen hat es mit sämtlichen verlusten in meinen leben, auf die ich mal alles gesetzt hab, es war einfach alles weg! Dann hat mich mal jemand gefragt, ob ich finde dass ich fett bin, da war ich allerdings NG irgendwie dachte ich, ja eigentlich stimmt es, ich kann mit vielen schlanken mädchen nicht mehr mithalten!
Also machte ich ne Diät!
Am anfang viel es mir nicht schwer das gewicht ging runter und ich freute mich, doch ich wollte stop machen, nicht mehr abnehmen, da ich dachte das wär langsam genug!

Doch dann stieß ich auf [auf die krankheitsverrlichenden Seiten], sie gaben mir unterstützung sie nahmen mich sofort bei ihnen aus, und ich hatte meine nächsten Erfolge! Dann wollt ich doch wieder aussteigen nach nem halben jahr, doch es ging einfach nicht, ich konnte nicht mehr essen ohne zu denken, wieviele kalos? was is da drin? wie verarbeitet es mein körper? wie lange dauert die verdauung? darf heut nichts mehr essen, nein, auf keinen fall!

Ich bekam in dieser zeit sehr oft FA's und kam damit nicht klar ich war in dieser Zeit schon UG doch nach den paar wochen FA's war ich genau an der kippe von UG zu NG und dann war ich auch wieder NG, und das war mir so zu doof, ich kehrte also wieder zurück!
Im sommer dann kam irgendwie der Große durchbruch für mich, ich hab wieder abgenommen und war eindeutig UG und mir gefiel es so sehr, ich wollte einfach weniger und noch weniger, weil immer wenn ich erfolge hatte wollte ich mehr!!!

Mittlerweile gehören mir zwei foren, und ich weiß nicht warum und was ich damit tun soll, irgendwie fühl ich mich für alle verantwortlich und sollte aus admiss auch irgendwie ein Vorbild sein, doch ich kann es einfach nicht!
Ich hab mir vorgenommen wenigstens nicht mehr Essenstagebücher aufzumachen und so doch vorgestern hab ich wieder eines eröffnet, und mich machts irgendwie fertig, wenn ich seh dass andere vl besser sein und mehr disziplin haben!
Ich bin mittlerweile schon "fast" NG aber ich kann das irgendwie nicht einsehen!!und ich will nicht so wirklich NG sein, ich hänge so sehr an meinem UG und wenn es wieder NG wird kommt es mir vor als hätt ich alles verloren? versteht ihr das?!

Und in der Schule gibts auch nur stress darüber, wisst ihr, meine freundinen, wollen mich zum Essen zwingen, oft fallen doofe sprüche, damit es auch die lehrer mitbekommen!

Ich weiß nicht mehr weiter, ich bin irgendwie extrem verwirrt und kann mit der Situation nicht umgehen!
Sorry wenn da jetzt auch müll drin steht, der was euch nicht interessiert, aber ich musste es irgendjemand sagen, und ich fühl mich ein stück besser und bin daher ner freundin dankbar die mich veranlasst hat, hier zu schreiben!!
Danke!

Doreen: quite unsure
Hi everyone! I'm not really sure if I'm in the right place, a friend advised me to write here, she is the only person that could have made me do something like this!
Good, to get to the point, I've been ["glamorizing anorexia"] for one year, but I'm not sure if that's right, and whether I'm really ill, or only want to be ill, I simply don't

know, personally I simply don't see it when someone says I'm ill or that I've got a problem!!

It began with the loss of everything in my life that I had pinned my hopes on, it was simply all gone! Then somebody asked me whether I think I'm fat, at that time I was actually normal weight somehow I thought, yes actually that's right, there are lots of thin girls I can't keep up with anymore.
So I went on a diet!
In the beginning I didn't find it difficult my weight dropped and I was happy, but I wanted to stop, not lose any more weight, because I thought it was getting to be enough. But then I stumbled across the [illness glamorizing websites], they supported me they accepted me immediately, and I went on to experience success!
Then after half a year I wanted to leave, but it just didn't work, I couldn't eat any more without thinking how many calos? what's in it? how will my body process it? how long will it take to digest? can't eat anything else today, no, on no account!

I binged a lot at that time and couldn't cope with it I was already underweight then but after a few weeks of binging I was exactly on the edge between underweight and normal weight and then I was normal weight again, and I found that too stupid, so I went back!
Then somehow in the summer came a big breakthrough for me, I had lost weight again and was clearly underweight and I liked it so much, I simply wanted less and less and even less, because whenever I had success I wanted more!!!

Since then I've taken charge of two forums, and I don't know why or what I should do with them, somehow I feel responsible for everything and as admiss I should somehow be a role model, but I just can't!
I resolved at least not to open any more food diaries and then the day before yesterday I did open one again, and somehow it kills me when I see that others are phps better and have more discipline!
In the meantime I'm "almost" normal weight again but I somehow can't accept that!!and I don't really want to be normal weight, I'm so very attached to being underweight and if the normal weight returns it seems to me as if I've lost everything? do you understand that?!

And at school there is only stress about it, you know, my friends want to force me to eat, often they come out with stupid comments so that the teachers can also hear them!

I don't know any more, I'm somehow extremely confused and can't deal with the situation!
Sorry if there's also rubbish in what I've written, stuff that doesn't interest you, but I had to tell someone, and I feel a bit better and therefore grateful to a friend that induced me to write here!!
Thank you!

In the opening of the thread, Doreen establishes herself as an insecure novice member, which is common (see chapter 6). The first sentence explains the insecurity as uncertainty about whether she is in the right place here, in the HO forum (line 1). Thus, the relevance of the location of explaining her problems is set, as well as the option for recipients to say that her contributions may be inappropriate *here*, in HO. Doreen marks what "the point" is, namely that she has been "glamorizing anorexia" for one year. The fashion in which she presents her pro-anorectic identity exhibits a problem orientation. On the one hand, by using part of the format for self-presentation (I have x since y years) the pro-ana identity is presented as fixed and involuntary as illnesses generally are. On the other hand, she adds: "But I am not sure whether that is right" (line 5-7), which implies moral accountability towards a voluntary, chosen identity. The word used by Doreen to categorize herself is not accepted by the moderator of the forum and is replaced by "glamorizing anorexia" (GA) (*magersuchtsverherrlichend*).[85] During the rest of the thread, further references to pro-ana made by both Doreen and other participants are replaced by the term "glamorizing illness" (*krankheitsverherrlichend*). Thus, the replacements made by the moderator (impossible to determine which moderator) are sanctions in reaction to violations of a certain HO rule related to language use. The topic as such is not prohibited, but just certain ways of labeling it. The fact that Doreen's posting is scrutinized and "corrected" increases the need to be extra cautious, about whether Doreen is actually "right here." In fact, it reveals something about her being there that is not quite right, namely, her word choice. This creates an atmosphere of controversy and taboo: There was something said that needed to be censored.

Line 5-7 point to the relevance of "the insight," mentioned in the introductory section above. According to Doreen, when somebody tells you that you are ill (or have a problem), the crucial issue is whether you see it yourself. Thus, reference to an insight emphasizes that eating problems are not just medically diagnosable illnesses, but also require a personal understanding (or insight) of the problem, or even an understanding of the self as being "ill." She reformulates the role of the insight in line 37, in which again

---

[85] It is very likely that Doreen originally used the term pro-ana, which stands for pro-anorexia. This term is probably erased to avoid instigation.

the relation between an objective fact (*fast "NG"*), and the connected insight are torn apart.

Throughout the first posting, Doreen seems to metaphorically embody the very concept of "glamorizing anorexia," which appears to be a collection of contradictions and paradoxes:

- Line 4-6: Being really ill or only wanting to be ill.
- Line 9-11: Being NG (normal weight) but agreeing that you are fat.
- Line 22-23: Being NG but finding that too silly.
- Line 25-26: Being UG (underweight) but perceiving it as a success.
- Line 35-36: Being NG means having lost everything.

These paradoxes are, in fact, only paradoxes in a context in which illness is understood as the agreement of bodily condition/medical diagnosis and personal insight, and in relation to this, wishing recovery, or the obligation to get well (cf. Parsons, 1951). This dimension is further analyzed in chapter 9. In this posting, health or recovery is also referred to as normal weight. When Doreen asks whether the HO members understand her (*versteht ihr das?!*, line 39), she points out the complexity, or paradoxical character of her problem through the combination of a question mark and an exclamation point. Furthermore, in line 44, she positions herself as extremely confused, and thus indirectly, as aware of the paradoxes she has articulated. She does not ask forum members to solve her problem, a puzzle of bodily facts (UG, etc.), attitudes (finding it silly) and desires (wanting to be ill). Rather, she expresses a certain gratitude for having had the opportunity to tell someone (line 46-48). This suggests that by typing the posting she got her sorrows "off her chest." The ending of the posting thus suggests that Doreen has not written in order to receive answers, but rather has used writing as a form of confessional cure. She calls recipients anybody (*irgendjemand*), as if it were unimportant who her readers are. The location of the forum (indexed with *hier*) has offered her the space to write, which is what Doreen is grateful for. The avoidance of directing a question or a wish towards the forum also secures her position towards the others: If she feels better after writing this posting, then criticizing the content would be unkind. The recycled invocation of the friend that made her post to HO in the first place (line 1 and line 47) helps to counter allegations that she may be in the wrong place. Since it was not her idea to post, her friend is ultimately responsible.

Paula welcomes and accepts Doreen on behalf of the forum as a member and does not go into the topic of pro-ana. Consider excerpt 15.

Excerpt 15 (#22) Continuation of excerpt 14

Paula (1)

46 erstmal Herzlich Willkommen bei HO!

47 Wenn du schon sagst das du an deinem UG hängst und es dir vorkommt als hättest du

48 alles verloren wenn du NG hast... Gesund ist das nicht. Du hast schonmal den ersten

49 Schritt gemacht dich hier anzumelden.

Paula (1)
firstly a Warm Welcome in HO!
If you already say that you are attached to being underweight and it seems to you as if you have lost everything when you have normal weight... That's not healthy. You've already taken the first step in registering here.

There are a few aspects of Paula's posting that seem significant with regard to the role of the community. Paula performs the almost standard welcome as a representative of the whole forum. As it was found in chapter 6, this can be analyzed as a response to the insecure openings. Secondly, note how *mal* (in both lines 1 and 2) in Doreen's posting is mirrored by *erstmal* preceding Paula's welcome. It renders the welcome the most essential part of the complete posting (because it is prioritized to the subsequent text), but also a part separate of the rest of the posting. First she offers her a welcome, in response to a novice member's posting, and she will then respond to the content of that specific posting. This prioritized welcome is indirectly an answer to the question of whether Doreen is "in the right place here," since it is a ritual through which Doreen is *erstmal* (which can also mean "conditionally," or "until further notice") accepted in HO. In this fashion it forestalls a reading of Doreen's insecurity as an insecurity that is related to the motivation to join HO. On the contrary, the welcome puts Doreen's doubt about becoming a member into the past tense; Doreen did not literally express that she pursues membership, but Paula's response makes her a member nonetheless.

In line 47-49, Paula deals with the paradoxical relation to illness sketched by Doreen. She does not, however, evaluate this relation directly, but uses various means to implicitly deliver her answer. First, she refers to what Doreen said herself (*Wenn du schon sagst*, line 47), which renders Doreen more accountable for what is to come, than Paula herself.[86] Second, she chooses one of Doreen's paradoxes. The if-then clause is not completed, since a "then" is not produced where the ellipsis appears. These suggest that the reader (Doreen) can guess what is to come. The complete clause could have been some-

[86] In other words, it can be characterized as an instance of "stake inoculation" (Potter, 1996).

something like: *If* you have already said that you would have lost everything if you were to be at a normal weight again, *then* it is clear that you have a problem. The then-clause in that case would have been a negative assessment of Doreen's condition. Instead, Paula produces a negatively formulated and thus indirect assessment: "That is not healthy" (*Gesund ist das nicht*, line 48). Notably, this formulation enables Paula to avoid directly saying that Doreen is ill, which is exactly what Doreen said she fails to see (line 5-7). On the other hand it is an explicit and univocal response to Paula's doubt. While Doreen's description of her condition was full of paradoxes, Paula's assessment is, though indirect, unambiguous: You are ill.

Paula describes Doreen's step to register for the forum as "the first step." She thus treats registering at the forum as an act of commitment, which is apparently linked not only to writing to the forum, but to "officially" registering, which is a precondition for participation (i.e., it is impossible to post without registering). This corresponds to the welcome, in which Paula already formally accepted Doreen as a novice member.

In this light, it is also worthwhile to compare the length of Doreen's and Paula's postings. Doreen, who used the posting to get trouble off her chest, typed a great deal of text, while Paula only briefly notes that Doreen has found the right place. Paula does not go into most of the issues raised by Doreen. It is as if Doreen is going through an intake session. She describes her problems at length and the expert (Paula on behalf of the forum) decides whether the help seeker can receive assistance at this forum. The answer is yes, the problem is recognized and Doreen is accepted, but the treatment itself has not yet started. The emoticon can be read both as a compliment for having had the courage to join HO and as encouragement that she should stay with HO and follow the path to recovery. In Doreen's subsequent reply to Paula's welcome she resists that the HO acceptance implies that she suddenly becomes *contra* eating disorders, see excerpt 16.

Excerpt 16 (#22) Continuation of excerpt 15.

Doreen (2)

50 danke das is lieb, hat mich gefreut dass sich jemand meldet, ich dachte wenn ich
51 schreib dass ich [krankheitsverherrlichend] bin, dass hier niemand antwortet, da alle
52 denken ich sei verrückt! ich weiß momentan echt nicht was tun! ich hab einfach angst
53 hier auch irgendwie zu versagen!
54 es war auch für mich nicht leicht mich hier anzumelden, ich denk ich hab ne gute
55 freundin gefunden die mir auf jedenfall den schubs in die richtige richtung gab, jetzt
56 hängt wohl alles von mir ab! aber ich kann jetzt noch nicht sagen, ob ichs schaff, und
57 durchziehen kann, aber ich will mir mal die chance geben es irgendwie zu ändern,
58 aber ich weiß es is sehr schwer, ich habs doch schon mal versucht und zwar alleine,

dieser versuch schlug damals fehl und ich hab versagt und ich hab furchtbare angst
dass es mir wieder passiert!!
danke dass ich hier sein kann!

Doreen (2)
thanks that's sweet, was happy somebody got in touch, i thought if i write that i'm [glamorizing illness], that nobody here would answer, then everybody would think i'm crazy! at the moment i really don't know what to do! i'm also simply frightened somehow of failing here!
it also wasn't easy for me to register here, i think i've found a good friend who definitely gave me a shove in the right direction, now it all depends on me! but i can't say yet whether i'll make it and can see it through, but i want to give myself a chance to change it somehow, but i know it's very difficult, i've already tried it once before and that was on my own, that attempt collapsed and i failed and i'm terribly frightened that it will happen to me again!!
thank you for giving me the chance to be here!

In the beginning of this posting, Doreen again performs her pro-anorectic identity and links this to her expectation that she would be ignored in HO because her identity would be considered crazy in HO. Why does she stress this? Positioning herself as pro-anorectic once more, after having been accepted in the "contra-community," works to resist that she would suddenly be contra now that she joined HO. Whereas Paula subtly included her in the contra-community, Doreen stresses that she is pro and at this point, she does not display any intention of abandoning this identity. However, she does change her word choice. Whereas in her first posting anorexia and UG were partly described as positive things (*Erfolge*, line 17, *Große durchburch*, line 27), in the second posting, Doreen, by contrast, alludes to attempts to recover from her eating disorder (*richtige richtung* line 55, *schaff* line 55, *versagt* line 59). She contends that she is in despair and fears failing here as well, which, in effect, makes a critique of her being pro-ana a "dispreferred" response (Pomerantz, 1984).

As Paula wrote on behalf of the forum (note that she did not reciprocally present herself), Doreen does not reply to Paula personally but to the whole forum. She is happy that *somebody* replied (line 50), feared that *nobody here* would respond, because *all* would think she was crazy (line 51-52) and that she has a fear of failing *here* too (line 58-59). Hence, the dialogue of these two members is more of a dialogue between a novice member and the HO forum in general, than between two individuals.

Consider line 54-56. Doreen again invokes her friend as the responsible party for her joining HO and thus repeatedly wards off any accountability for joining. This is a denial of what Paula said, namely that registration for

HO was the first step. Put differently, Doreen does not display a willingness to see her fresh membership of HO as her own success: Due to her friend she is now in HO, but she is not at all sure whether she will make it. She is standing on HO's doorstep and is terrified that she will fail in HO, since she has failed already in a previous attempt. Despite her not subscribing to HO's contra-eating disorders position and the enormous fear of failure, Doreen thanks HO for accepting her (line 60). Paula replies to both aspects. Consider excerpt 17.

Excerpt 17 (#22) Continuation of excerpt 16.

Paula (2)

60 Hier kann man nicht versagen!
61 Aber lass die Finger von [den krankheitsverrlichenden Seiten], das ist doch der totale
62 Wahnsinn...

Paula (2)
It's not possible to fail here!
But keep away from the [glamorizing illness sites], that's just total madness...

Paula does explicitly criticize pro-anorexia, however, without excluding Doreen from HO on those grounds. She first delivers the preferred response to Doreen's fear of failure by stating that, in general, it is impossible to fail in HO. This works to reassure Doreen, which is again formulated not as a personal comfort, but as a general characteristic of HO, which she presents on behalf of the forum's members. However, in the next sentence, she describes pro-anorectic websites as total insanity (*totale Wahnsinn*, line 61-62). This implies that visiting these sites is not considered failing in HO; rather, these websites are beyond intelligibility, beyond reason.

How does Paula get her critical message across without dismissing Doreen as a novice member? She avoids discussing the pro-identity but does refer to the act of visiting pro-ana websites. In other words, the identity (seemingly fixed and involuntary) is turned into an action, which is a construction that calls for personal accountability that is even clearer than a pro-ana identity. The point is not that Doreen is accountable for her problem, but that Paula's formulation as an alternative description of Doreen's problem increases Doreen's self-responsibility. Simultaneously, this alternative, action-focal description of the problem simplifies Doreen's problem. Just leaving these pro-ana websites aside seems to be less difficult than switching one's identity from pro to contra.

In sum, the dialogue between Doreen and Paula can best be described as the knock on HO's door by a controversial, pro-anorectic novice member, the subsequent acceptance by HO regardless of her controversial identity, and the eventual univocal indication that pro-ana is wrong, without dismissing her.

The next contributor, Food, applies a different strategy, namely a personal rather than a community approach.

Excerpt 18 (#22) Continuation of excerpt 17.

Food (1)

Hallo Süße, schön dass du hier bist und es geschafft hast! Bist mir sehr wichtig und ich finds klasse dass du schonmal einen schritt in eine zumindest andere richtung als [weiter die Krankheit zu veherrlichen] gemacht hast. ich weiß aus – leider – eigener erfahrung, dass es total schwer ist zu verstehen, dass die die einen immer unterstützen und einem scheinbar helfen [auf den krankheitsverrlichenden Seiten] im grunde keine echten freunde sein können, da sie nicht das beste für einen wollen: gesundheit. sie ermuntern einen ja bloß zum sichkaputthungern. Viele wissen auch nicht wirklich oder wollen es nicht wissen, dass sie krank sind, da sie MS mit Untergewicht gleichsetzen und wenn sie NG sind denken sie wären nicht krank. das zu erkennen dauert eine Zeit, gerade wenn man pro ist, aber aus eigenem antrieb zumindest mal daran zu zweifeln find ich sehr mutig, es ist schließlich einfacher in der anderen community zu bleiben, dann muss man nicht gegen die ES kämpfen und man hat (scheinbar) freunde, die einen "verstehen".

Aber Maus, auch hier verstehen einen die Leute, auch wenn sie nicht pro sind und dass du an der Bewegung zweifelst ist ein großer Schritt, ich hoffe für dich dass du Abstand dazu gewinnen und es vielleicht irgendwann loslassen kannst um FÜR DICH zu kämpfen, du bist es wert und mir wichtig, weil du mich in den letzten Tagen auch ganz lieb abgelenkt hast und man mit dir super reden kann. Also bitte mach weiter so, ich brauch dich noch 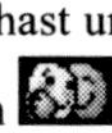LG

Food (1)

Hello Sweetie, it's great that you're here and have made it! You're very important to me and I think it's excellent that you've already taken a step in at least another direction from [continuing to glamorize the illness]. i know – unfortunately – from personal experience that it's really difficult to understand, that those who always support us and apparently help [on the glamorizing illness sites] basically can't be real friends, because they don't want the best for us: good health. they only encourage us to starveourselvestodeath. Many also don't really know or don't want to know that they are ill, because they equate anorexia with being underweight and if they have normal weight they think they aren't ill. it takes some time to recognize that, especially if one is pro, but i find it very brave to at least have doubts about it of your own

accord, in the end it's easier to stay in the other community because then you don't have to fight against the ED and you have friends (apparently) that "understand" you.
But Mouse, the people here also understand us, even if they're not pro and that you're having doubts about the movement is a big step, i hope for you that you can distance yourself and perhaps at some point let go in order to fight FOR YOURSELF, you are worth it and important to me, because you have diverted me very sweetly in the last few days and it's possible to really talk to you. So please keep it up, I still need you 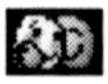 *Love*

Food attempts to keep Doreen "on board" by criticizing the pro-community and stressing that she needs Doreen in HO (*eigener Erfahrung*, line 64, *du bist es wert und mir wichtig*, line 76-77, *ich brauch dich noch*, line 78).[87] Throughout the posting, the pro-community is not depicted as an identity (being pro), but rather as a social alliance (*community*, line 72, *Bewegung*, line 75) and there is no doubt about its quality (though it is not described as unintelligible [cf. *Wahnsinn*]):

1. In the pro-community, you will not find any *real* friends.
2. In the pro-community, they do not strive for your best (= health).
3. In the pro-community, they do not know or refuse to recognize that they are ill.
4. In the pro-community they are confused about the relation between normal weight (NG) and illness (Food claims that being NG does not mean someone is not ill, line 69-70).

In contrast to Paula, Food does not describe Doreen's registration as the first step to recovery, but as having achieved something (*geschafft*, line 62). She mitigates "the first step" to a step in at least a different direction than pro-ana (*einen schritt in eine zumindest andere richtung als*, line 63). This implies that the dichotomy between pro and contra communities has been somewhat relaxed, or at least that distancing oneself from pro does not entail that one is contra. Indirectly, this position is a critique of Paula's postings, in which being in HO was equated with being contra, and pro was depicted as total insanity.

[87] Line 77-78 of this posting suggests that Food and Doreen have had forum contact before, at least during the past days (*weil du mich in den letzten Tagen ganz lieb abgelenkt hast*). Therefore, we cannot conclude that this extreme display of intimacy and closeness (ordinarily only acted out between people who know each other to a certain extent) is, in HO, also common between strangers.

The following contribution comes from Eleanor, who uses yet another strategy in dealing with the pro-anorectic novice member. She avoids treating pro and contra as a clear opposition and Doreen as already a member of HO; instead she challenges her to become a member.

Excerpt 19 (#22) Continuation of excerpt 18.

Eleanor (1)

Hallo, schön, dass du hier bist!

Ich finde es wichtig dass sich beide Seiten nicht bekriegen, egal ob verherrlichende oder dagegen. Deshalb würde ich es auch nicht so kritisch beurteilen, dass du hier zu HO gekommen bist, denn im Grunde geht es auf beiden Arten von Seiten um ähnliches: wir wollen um unsere Ängste, Sorgen und Probleme mit uns, der Gesellschaft und den andern reden und Verständnis finden – finde ich zu mindest. Das wichtige hier ist, wie du selbst ja auch schreibst, dass wir uns hier nicht vergleichen müssen, wetteifern müssen um einen Status, der realistisch betrachtet den Tod bedeutet. jeder der hier ist möchte versuchen ein halbwegs normales Leben zu führen. Finde es schön, dass du neugierig darauf geworden bist und hier her guckst!

Mach dir mal keine Gedanke um deinen Status als Admiss. Der Vorschlag die Foren zu schließen ist hier wohl etwas übereilt – kommt evtl. ja irgendwann von dir selbst! Nimm dir da lieber erst mal den Stress, nimm dich einfach raus ... die Leute kommen auch ganz gut miteinander zurecht. Außerdem steht doch nicht einer im Mittelpunkt, an dem sich alle messen ... also ich kann mir nicht vorstellen, dass sich die anderen mit nur mit dir vergleichen und sich ihren Teil denken, wenn du nicht ins Bild passt. Nimm dir echt einfach mal ne Auszeit und versuche dich zu orientieren ... einfach mal spüren, was du willst! Wenns dir nicht taugt: zurück kannst du immer, aber sich auf was neues und anderes einzulassen kostet Mut! Bist du mutig?

Eleanor

Hello, it's great that you're here!

I find it important that both sides are not at war with each other, whether they glamorize or are against that. Therefore I wouldn't judge it as so critical that you've come here to HO, because the two sides are basically about the same thing: we want to talk to and be understood by ourselves, society and the others about our fears, worries and problems – at least I think so. The important thing, as you write yourself, is that we don't have to compare ourselves here, compete with each other for status, which looked at realistically means death. everybody here wants to try to lead a reasonably normal life. Find it great that you have become inquisitive about it and are looking this way!

Don't worry about your status as admiss. The suggestion to shut down the forums is certainly overhasty – it may happen eventually by itself! Rather don't stress yourself, simply get yourself out of there ... those people get on really well with each other. Moreover, nobody is standing in the center with everybody measuring themselves up against them... so I can't imagine that the others compare themselves with only with you and are quietly critical if you don't fit into the picture. Just simply take some time out for yourself and try to get some orientation ... simply get a feel for what you want! If it's no good: you can always go back, but to venture out into something new requires bravery! Are you brave?
Eleanor

Eleanor initially reconciles pro- and contra-communities (pro-ana and HO) as if they were more similar than different. Eventually HO membership is constructed as something that requires courage, which means that she treats Doreen's first posting not as someone who has already found that courage but rather as a non-committal observing in HO. Thereby, she does not only respond to Doreen, but indirectly to both Paula and Food as well. She first states that she would not critically judge whether Doreen has come to HO, implying that others (Paula) have. She defines what the two sides have in common: We want to talk about our fears, sorrows and problems with ourselves, the society and others and come to an understanding about them. The special thing about HO is that you do not have to compete for status which could actually lead to death. It is notable that Eleanor denies that this peculiar detail of HO is *essentially* different, because she does indicate that HO prevents a practice that could ultimately lead to death (competition), which the pro-community does not prevent.

Second, Eleanor counters the idea that HO members, by being contra eating disorders, are on their way to becoming normal. Instead, she circumscribes the engagement of each HO member as trying to lead a "halfway" normal life (line 85-86). She thus avoids categorizing eating disorders in terms of an ill-normal dichotomy of health. From this perspective, HO members do not see themselves as ill people who strive to become normal. The point is not being ill or normal but trying to lead a sort of normal life. Third, she does not speak of Doreen's first step (unlike Paula), or a step that could at least be perceived as being in a different direction (like Food), but minimizes Doreen's registration at HO even further by stating: "It is nice that you have become curious and that you are having a look around here" (*Finde es schön, dass du neugierig darauf geworden bist und hier her guckst*, line 86-87). Eleanor advises Doreen to take her time and keep her distance (from the pro-community) before making up her mind about what she wants (line 93-94). Hence, she does not treat Doreen as a HO member just yet. Instead, she constructs Doreen's first contributions as looking around in HO, without having really decided if she wants to become a member of this community. Eleanor refers to a personal orientation or feeling, which is comparable to the insight (*versuche dich zu orientieren…einfach mal spüren, was du willst!*, line 94). She stresses that it requires bravery to become involved in HO, and by challenging Doreen to have the courage she treats Doreen as someone who is not yet a member. This can be seen as a response to the fact that Doreen repeatedly pointed out that it was a friend who encouraged to contribute, and that it was not of her own volition. Finally, two very brief postings form the closing of the thread, see excerpt 20.

Excerpt 20 (#22) Continuation of excerpt 19.

Doreen (3)
mal danke an alle! ihr seid echt süß und irgendwie bin ich froh dass ich mal hier schreiben konnte, tat gut!
und @eleanor, ich weiß nicht ob ich mutig bin, wirklich nicht, aber ich werds versuchen!
danke nochmal an alle 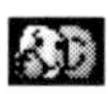

Food (2)
konnte?
weitermachen...! 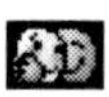

Doreen (3)
thank you to everyone! u r really sweet and somehow i'm happy that i could write here, did me good!
and @eleanor, i don't know whether i'm brave, i really don't, but i will try to be!
thank's again to everybody 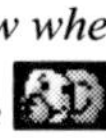

Food (2)
could?
keep it up…! 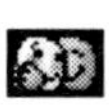

In her last posting, posted the next day, Doreen refers to writing in HO and how it has worked for her in the past tense. She responds to Eleanor personally about being unsure about whether she has the courage, which suggests that she does not immediately take up the challenge, but perhaps just needs more time.

Two aspects suggest that Doreen has declined HO membership. First, by thanking everyone (probably referring to respondents Paula, Food and Eleanor) not only at the start of this posting, but again at the end, she does not do anything to keep the conversation going. The "thank you" functions as a closing remark (compare: Thank you, bye bye). The hug offered through the emoticon functions to mitigate the declination. Second, Food's reply (line 102-103), which expresses encouragement (both verbally and figuratively through a hug), displays a reading of Doreen's posting as "giving up." In other words, she reads Doreen's posting as a declination of membership.

However, Doreen initiates threads in other HO sub-forums on the same day, in which she does not reveal her pro-identity. In fact, during the subsequent eighteen months, she opens threads and contributes to various discussions. In other words, what seemed to be a declination was not actually so. Nevertheless, implicitly declining serves to dodge accountability for a controversial, pro-ana identity.

8.7 Conclusion

It is noteworthy that various novices who have asked the "diagnostic" question of whether they are still normal or ill, are not offered a response. This is noteworthy, since the HO forum was also set up for those who are still living in isolation with their problems and have thus never been diagnosed before. The question can therefore be described as legitimate, but is not quite treated as such in HO.

In two cases, the question or issue of being ill is (in)directly touched upon by respondents. The two threads initiated by Sylvia and Doreen can be considered forum conversations in which the limits of forumability are explored. The interest of the novices can be described as becoming accepted in the HO community, despite ambivalence about it. Their recipients are peers who share similar problems with the novice, which leads to the expectation that s/he will be taken seriously and does not need to account for the illness as interviewees may feel compelled to in an interview situation. It appeared, however, that the illness was not always recognized by novices. They expressed doubt about whether they were ill as a result of the degree or absence of certain symptoms. Whereas others constructed their illness as a fact (through a diagnosis), these newcomers "oriented to" scales, degrees, presence or absence of symptoms, etc., which led them to suppose that their conditions could still be normal. Hence, these novice members did not or cannot enact an eating disorder identity, which appeared to be the admission ticket to the forum (chapter 7).

However, novice members who do not present their eating behaviors and the conditions of their bodies as univocally ill exhibit this as problematic themselves, by saturating their postings with paradoxes and with markers of what is generally known about being "ill" (e.g., underweight). At the same time, also recipients orient to this ambivalence towards illness as a problem, but they offer various solutions. Either limits of forumability are set clearly (Marcia by defining that being in HO is knowing that you are ill, and Paula by treating HO membership as the first step to recovery), or forumability also incorporates the not (yet) unambiguous articulation of the insight and the related desire and intention to get well (Jennifer and Joe, Food and Eleanor). This means that the normative requirement of doing being eating disordered is not as strict as it may have seemed in the previous chapter. However, these positions or opinions about the limits of forumability are not equally strong when we compare the two extensive case studies. In the first case (Sylvia's thread in section 8.5), it is a moderator who has the last word. Her authority sanctions the novice by not leaving any doubt about what the forum stands for, with the (apparent) consequence that the novice is rejected as a member. In the second case (section 8.6), the forum is implicitly defined in three alternative ways (as radically excluding pro, as contra but leaving room for those who convert, and those who are not definable through the pro/contra dichotomy), but it seems that none of them are accepted by the novice, at least not overtly. The question of acceptance by the community is turned into a question of courage on the part of the novice (Eleanor's posting treats Doreen as not-yet-a-member, and points her to the courage it requires to get into the community). This implies that HO membership is involved with having a personal conviction, insight or readiness, which is not necessarily, or not solely, related to symptoms or body weight.

The insight that you are ill can also be displayed by the recognition of being a candidate for therapy. With this recognition one is not expected to actually engage in therapy; there are other reasons or barriers not to (cf. Joe who fears that *as a man* he would not be taken serious by a medical practitioner). Therapy for pro-ana is never mentioned. Eleanor does not depict HO participation as the first step toward recovery or treatment. She prefers to foreground the intention of HO members (and possibly pro-community members as well) to lead a halfway normal life, which is not fatal. This position is rarely advanced in the HO forum, but it seems to suggest that self-regulation (i.e., not seeking medical treatment) is also an option for dealing with an eating disorder. This position however, does not seem to be accepted when it is proposed by novice members (cf. Sylvia). In all of these cases, the main and minimum requirement for novice members is that they somehow display the insight that they are ill.

Part III

Interpretation and conclusion

Chapter 9

Entering the online support group and adopting the sick role

The empirical analysis has yielded insight into the relevancies of the initial phases of online community membership. It seems that new members are usually cordially accepted, if they have presented themselves as legitimate members. A diagnosis or variant (e.g., underweight) suffices to display legitimacy. However, it also became clear that in the case of less univocal admissions (centering on the question "am I ill?"), normative requirements concerning membership are communicated, either indirectly or even rather explicitly. The norm appears to be that members admit that they are ill.

In the last part of this thesis, I offer an interpretation of these findings regarding illness behavior and its potentially specific developments in relation to the occurrence of online support groups, drawing on sick role theory (Parsons, 1951). The social expectations tied to illness can be considered the background knowledge that participants use as a resource to account for their actions. The relevance of the early stages of illness, as they are discerned in further developments of sick role theory, is mainly useful for an understanding of the process of entering an online support group.

9.1 The sick role from an interpretive perspective

Since the birth of medical sociology, illness is no longer considered as merely a biological or medical issue, but also something that plays an important role in society (Gerhardt, 1989). Parsons (1939) was the first to consider medical practice as a social system in its own right. He viewed illness as more than a physical or mental condition, namely as constitutive of a social role, which is defined as the failure to fulfill other social roles in a normal way (Parsons, 1951). The ethnomethodological critique of this type of theory is the implicit assumption that subjects are "cultural dopes" that simply adopt the roles designed for them (Garfinkel, 1967). Nevertheless, sick role theory can be used to explain some of the relevancies for participants of online support groups.

The functionalist concept of the sick role implies the norms that people need to understand in order to participate in a specific situation. The interaction between doctors and patients is structured in precise detail by the predefined norms of behavior for people playing the roles. From a functionalist perspective, these roles are essential in order for the health-care system to function adequately and smoothly.

Parsons claimed that the sick role requires legitimacy, which means that it is related to certain social norms. Legitimacy is secured when certain norms are obeyed. He discerned several aspects, which are related to the sick role and its demand for legitimization, generally summarized as two rights and two duties (e.g., Segall, 1976). The rights encompass the lack of individual responsibility for the condition and the exemption from "normal" social role responsibilities (e.g., work and care), depending on the nature and severity of the illness. The duties concern the obligation to try to get well and the expectation that the sick person will seek and accept technically competent help and cooperate with the physician. This implies the patient's recognition of diagnosis and compliance with treatment, unless there are appropriate reasons to doubt the received treatment.[88] For a discussion of norms relevant to the sick role, I focus on Parsons' formulated duties rather than rights. We may assume that not living up to the duties should be understood as norm-breaking behavior, which may lead to sanctioning.

From an interpretive perspective, the duties must be considered norms that members can "orient to" in order to create and sustain a particular definition of the situation. In the course of conduct, they come to perceive each other as playing a certain role, rather than some other possible role. This implies a concept of norms that are observable in the participants' interpretation of prior actions, or projections of a future action, in which the process of interpretation always mediates between action and norm. Various members can perform different actions in response to a norm relevancy, which means that norms are not viewed as fixed and prescriptive, but more as resources for social interaction instead.

The basis of norms lies in background knowledge and expectations. Actors should be seen as having acquired a body of normatively organized knowledge in terms of which they treat their own and one another's actions as accountable (Garfinkel, 1967; Heritage, 1984). Socially shared knowledge is among other things condensed into categories, category-bound features and the categories' inferences (Schegloff, 2007). However, the focus of an interpretive study is not on this normative, shared knowledge itself, but rather on actors' forms of conduct as orientations to this knowledge. The motivation to

[88] In later system-theoretical thinking (e.g., Luhmann, 1990), the system of medical care is still in correspondence with Parsons' definition of the sick role, as it is still centered on the ill-healthy dichotomy and the doctor-patient relationship, in which the doctor is the one who declares the patient healthy.

act normatively appropriate is tailored by the actor's awareness of the differential accountability of alternative courses of conduct. The term normative requirement (rather than duty) thus refers to the reflexive projection of a normatively appropriate action in the ad hoc situation. This means that normative requirements are understood as participants' local interpretations of what is required.

Hence, from an interpretive/ethnomethodological point of view, illness incumbency is an intersubjective and situational accomplishment, rather than merely constituting a predefined or predictable role (Gerhardt, 1989). The sick role's norms can be seen as shared knowledge that members somehow "orient to," rather than as *prescribing* normative role behavior. Thus, the norms and expectations related to illness are observable implicitly in accounts: The member that delivers the account has interpreted the situation in such a way that a specific illness norm was relevant there. This means that accounts make an action retrospectively recognizable as something unusual or troublesome. Thus, they clarify what the action supposedly is and has always been. However, the occurrence of an account does not necessarily infer a norm debilitation. Rather, accounts "prevent conflicts from arising by verbally bridging the gap between action and expectation" (Scott and Lyman, 1968: 46). However, according to Scott and Lyman (1968), one of the limits to this peacekeeping function is that background expectations (i.e., taken-for-granted knowledge concerning, for instance, illness), should not be violated. This means that accounts enable members to prevent disputes, unless they violate background expectations. Thus, if accounts concerning illness are not accepted, apparently some basic illness norm is relevant.

9.2 Further developments of the sick sole

Before I interpret some of the findings of the discourse analysis from the sick role perspective, a few further developments in sick role theory need to be explained. The sick role definition is a *theoretical* concept and thus defines the "ideal-type" of role; it does not provide an empirical measurement of the concepts' reality. In the decades since Parsons' studies on the sick role, numerous empirical studies have discovered aspects of both the nature of the illness and its social context that require modifications and extensions of the sick role to make it empirically (more) valid (Segall, 1976). For instance, chronic illness, terminal conditions, aging and pregnancy require modifications with regard to the assumption of the temporary nature of illness and the striving for a cure. It was also revealed that the psychiatric sick role differs substantially from the medical one (Segall, 1976). Two aspects seem crucial in the modification of the psychiatric sick role:

- Conditions with a psychological component or connotation make the question of personal responsibility, which is related to the stigma of mental illness relevant. Nevertheless, the individual is expected to try to get well and seek professional help.
- The psychiatric role does not demand the passiveness of the patient in relation to the doctor, but rather, s/he is expected to be active, independent and self-directed in her/ his interactions with the doctor.

Even with these adaptations, the duties of trying to get well and seeking competent help also seem valid for the modified sick role for psychiatric conditions.

Sick role theory has also been further developed in yet another direction, since the ill person experiences a process of actually adopting the social role of sickness. This process is intertwined with the step that involves seeking professional help. Mechanic (1978) expanded sick role theory with a theory of help-seeking behavior in which the perception or definition by the individual of the situation at hand and the ability of the individual to cope with the situation serve as the two central factors. In this way, Mechanic's advancement of sick role theory explains that the individual's perceptions and decisions play an important role in the period before the sick role is actually adopted.

In accordance with this, it has been observed that there are various stages of illness behavior (Suchman, 1965):

- The symptom experience stage
- The assumption of the sick role stage
- The medical care contact stage
- The dependent patient stage
- The recovery or rehabilitation stage.

Suchman's (1965) first stage of illness coincides with some of the variables Mechanic discerns (e.g., the extent to which the symptoms are perceived as serious or dangerous [Mechanic, 1978]). This implies that self-observation has been viewed as an important stage in (or directly prior to) the adoption of the sick role.

In the following section, I will show that the study of HO interactions confirms that becoming a member of an online support group can be adequately described as the relevancy of the sick role, including its stages and norms.

9.3 The online support group and the sick role

The study has revealed that the first postings to an online support group are composed, on the one hand, by members who present themselves as new to the forum and/or new to the issue of eating disorders, and, on the other hand, by members who have a long experience with eating disorders and/or the forum. These two types of members relate to the sick role in different ways.

Newcomers treat the step of entering a community as a step in the direction of adopting the sick role. The uncertainty and hesitancy observed in the newcomers' first postings could be interpreted as having some doubt about whether their symptoms are actually serious enough to seek help and assume the sick role (e.g., chapter 7 excerpts 9, 12 and 13 and chapter 8 excerpt 11). However, the insecurity also points to a difficulty inherent in this phase, which may be linked to the threat of stigmatization. The novice members' ambivalence towards joining the community can thus be explained as a reluctance toward actually adopting the sick role.

The ways that regular members deal with this reluctance works in two directions. Through their generosity of welcoming and complementing they emphasize that the newcomer is now a member of the community (e.g., chapter 6 excerpt 19 and chapter 8 excerpt 15). In this way, they assist the newcomer in adopting the sick role. A newcomer who fears social stigmatization is reassured, because by being a member of a group, the stigma is at the very least shared by the rest of the members. Community membership thus implies adoption of the sick role, since it is viewed as help-seeking behavior and seeking help implies the recognition that you are ill. The sick role's normative requirement to pursue a cure is then lived up to.

However, a newcomer who presents her/himself as a person in the first stage of the sick role is not sure whether the symptoms s/he observes are actually serious enough to be described as ill. This type of newcomer may not strive for community membership as long as s/he is uncertain about her/his condition. Therefore, s/he may express ambivalence about community membership, because s/he is not willing or ready to actually adopt the sick role (chapter 8). In this case, the acceptance by experienced members as a member of the community is premature and does not offer much space for members in the earliest stage of the sick role.

Sufferers who have already been diagnosed, or those who have been active in the forum before, can be characterized as being in the third and fourth stages of the sick role. They immediately present themselves as occupants of the sick role by communicating their diagnosis. Diagnoses display the result of a professional consultation, and thus indirectly seem to show that the individual has lived up to the sick role's norms with regard to the pursuit of cure.

These entries are basically unproblematic; the novices are smoothly accepted as members of the community. In these cases, the online support group is treated as additional support to professional treatment. Hence, in the case of online support groups the requirement to seek out professional help is relaxed to the obligation to use the online service as supportive of self-help.

Even ex-sufferers initiate threads in the New Here sub-forum. They may have already recovered from the illness, but may experience a relapse and therefore want to "re-enter" the forum. By presenting themselves as ex-sufferers they define themselves in the last stage of the sick role.

Members "orient to" the norm of wanting to get well and of seeking assistance (the duties of the sick role). They offer accounts for why they joined the forum, which emphasize that they expect to find help, support or strength in community membership. The fact that they mainly seek help and support for their project of self-help confirms that the psychiatric role demands that the patient is active in her/his recovery process.

Thus, in various regards the sick role's norms seem to be as relevant in online support groups as they are in other components of the medical system, although the project of self-help is probably more important here. In this regard, people who join an online support group are confronted with the sick role's norms as a "set of institutionalized expectations and the corresponding sentiments and sanctions" (Parsons, 1951: 436), at least they draw on these expectations in their communicative actions despite the fact that they do not find themselves in a medical institution.

However, the study has revealed a few aspects that do seem to conflict with the general sick role's norms. First, newcomers are not immediately confronted with the responsibility of seeking professional help. For some sufferers, this would be experienced as a threat. In the online support group HO, medical treatment is recommended (chapter 6 excerpt 9), but not required for membership. The relaxation of the general sick role's duty renders the online support group substantially more approachable than the doctor.

Second, some members assert that they perceive (or previously perceived) the symptom of being underweight as success or as something desirable, which conflicts with the recognition that one is ill and thus breaks with the norm of trying to get well (chapter 8 excerpt 7). Similarly, some members break with the norm of trying to get well by expressing sympathy for the pro-ana movement that views the illness as an admirable lifestyle (chapter 8 excerpt 14).

Nevertheless, it would be indefensible to characterize the online support group as a social realm, which defies the sick role's norms. This is mainly because experienced members try to direct the newcomers toward the general sick role norms. This means that claims that have violated certain norms will be responded to with a call for further explanation. If the newcomer can convincingly account for the norm debilitation (e.g., "I am not sure myself", chapter 8 excerpt 14), the newcomer will still be allowed to join the community. The most plausible explanation for this relaxation of norms is probably that regulars recognize this behavior as typical for the early stages of the sick role. The newcomer is experiencing symptoms (stage 1) but does not yet recognize them as serious enough. S/he may sometimes even experience symptoms as satisfying (such as weight loss). In other words, s/he may still need some time to actually assume the sick role (stage 2). The online support group seems to offer a space to discuss one's thoughts and feelings concerning these early stages. Regular members tolerate certain anormative formulations, because they view them as typical of "first stage" sufferers. However, it is striking that frequently they do not respond to or go into explicit questions about (degrees of) illness and normality (section 8.4). Hence, the newcomer is accepted without receiving an answer to the question whether s/he is really ill. It seems that being allowed into the community stands for an affirmative answer: "You are ill." However, whether this is really the case or whether this actually helps newcomers to adopt the sick role is questionable.

9.4 The importance of the early stages

It has been suggested that the early stages of illness, which involve self-observation, have become increasingly important recently. It has been argued that the question of illness (which is central in these stages) has shifted from a dichotomy (health-illness) to a scale. According to Hahn (2003), contemporary health has become a totalizing principle, which rejects the view that diagnosis is simply tied to health and illness codes, which are linked to the medical system:

> *Gesundheit ist wie Wirtschaft, Recht, Wissenschaft oder Liebe eine totalisierende Perspektive geworden, unter der alles und jedes jederzeit zum Thema werden kann.* (Hahn, 2003: 32).
>
> [Health is like economics, law, science and love; it has become a totalizing principle, which means it can broach any issue at any time.]

He believes this development is related to the rise of normalism (Link, 1999).[89] Nowadays, people are faced with the task of self-observation, self-

[89] According to Link (1999), normalism is a specifically modern phenomenon of westernized societies, which has beomce particularly consolidated over the last few decades (since 1968). It refers to the selectively strategic use of statistics by the insurance industry (*Ver-Sicherung*) and the redistribution (*Um-Verteilung*) of

control, and paying attention as well as ensuring the care for their own normality. The responsibility for self-control and self-diagnosis is high, especially with regard to health issues. As a result, the sick role has become detached from the health-illness dichotomy as it was thought by both Parsons (1951) and Luhmann (1990), and replaced by a continuum of health and illness, based on values of normality, on which individuals position themselves. The relevant question is then no longer centered on the codes ill/healthy, but on the differential of beneficial (*dienlich*) or harmful (*abträglich*) to one's health (Hahn, 2003: 32).

The present study confirms this observation of change, mainly with regard to the self-observation of symptoms. Members formulate doubt about the normality of their behavior or body, unless they have already consulted a medical professional who has categorized them as ill.

It is striking that members often use medical terminology to describe their symptoms. In HO, the Body Mass Index (BMI) is frequently used in the process of self-observation. The BMI is a tool used to decide an individual's normality in terms of weight. It is, however, still considered a controversial tool (Wirtz, 2008). It indicates whether a person is underweight, normal or overweight. The BMI is often used to determine anorexia nervosa and therefore plays an important role in clinical practice. However, in HO, members describe themselves in terms of BMI measurement concepts: overweight, normal weight and underweight (typically through abbreviations), using adjectives to express degrees of underweight.[90] In other words, medical concepts are applied for lay observations. Although the terminology suggests that the person may have received medical care, it appears that describing symptoms in medical terms does not mean that the person recognizes and has adopted the sick role in a social setting. It is not uncommon for newcomers of an online support group to use medical concepts in their self-descriptions (cf. Lamerichs, 2003), however, it is striking that in HO the medically "ill" label of underweight does not warrant that members admit that they are ill.

---

progress. The "product" of this phenomenon is normality. It reveals itself both in scientific discourses (*Spezialdiskurse*) and in "interdiscursive" contexts, such as everyday life practices and discourses.

[90] It must be emphasized that members may also wish to offer kilogram and length details, but also calories and descriptions of food portions, but this is not permitted in HO to avoid comparisons among members (see 4.2).

9.5 Peer support and the sick role

The relevance of the early stages of illness in the first interactions in the online support group reveals an important role for peers. In the traditional concept of the sick role the main part is played by the medical practitioner, while in the online support group, illness is the chief topic of negotiation *among peers*. The patient-patient relationship must therefore be recognized as a highly important factor in illness behavior in addition to the doctor-patient relationship. The sick role as a concept, according to McKay (2001), does not sufficiently account for this, since it over-represents the biomedical perspective on illnesses. Current understandings of illness in general are shifting away from medical practitioners and towards patients (e.g., Frank, 1994), who no longer accept the passivity implied in the sick role. McKay has argued that patients' illness narratives, as presented in books, TV shows, magazines, but also online support groups, are evidence of this change. The Internet has to a large extent enabled the possibility of engaging in peer interactions in the absence of doctors.[91] Hence, it seems necessary to recognize increased patient activity in illness behavior. This is both related to self-observation and self-diagnosis and to the increasing discussion about these self-observations among peers (enabled by, among other things, the rise of online support groups).[92]

However, the social norms relevant to the sick role, which are institutionalized expectations as Parsons formulated them, have not been fundamentally rejected and replaced by alternative understandings and norms by the patient groups, but have generally been adopted and, in some situations, slightly relaxed.

9.6 Explaining the relaxation of norms: Sociability

The study showed that norm-breaking behavior was tolerated for the early stages of the sick role, but not actually approved. Hence, the way in which respondents react to novices who, for instance, report feelings of success concerning underweight, indicates that the breaking with background expectations of what is normative behavior is to a certain extent tolerated or ig-

[91] It is likely that the young, higher educated urbanites are using the Internet for health communication more than others. This is, at least, the case in the US (Rains, 2008).

[92] Increased self-diagnosis and increased attention being paid to patients' illness experiences have another consequence: Sufferers have also become collectively (and thus politically) more active in the sense that they organize themselves and collectively fight for changes in medical practice (e.g., women with attention deficit disorder [Liebsch, 2007]).

nored because another interactional cause is prioritized. Respondents thus refrain from calling for an account, which does not mean that they promote the breaking of norms. Scott and Lyman have explained this phenomenon as follows:

> Under certain situations behavior that would ordinarily require an account is normalized without interruption or any call for an account. Typically such situations are social conversations in which the values to be obtained by the total encounter supersede those which would otherwise require excuses or justifications (1968: 55).

According to them, one of these values is sociability. Participants would refrain from calling for an account of this norm-breaking behavior, because the total encounter has another value, which is more important than the accountability issue. This other value is social in character. This seems to adequately describe the actions of both novices and respondents in the HO community: The core relevance of the sub-forum for novice members is the activity of becoming a member by presenting the self and being welcomed. Here, the situation's focus is social rather than medical or illness-related. Respondents in their replies do point out how to interpret the novices' norm-breaking descriptions in a normative fashion. They, for instance, explain that feelings of success after weight loss or the desire for (more) weight loss are, in fact, symptoms of the illness. Another example is that, in response to postings in which the expectation to try to get well is not lived up to, the novice is recommended to do therapy (e.g., chapter 8 excerpt 9). These are not clearly instances of sanctioning, but more subtle responses to norm-breaking behavior. Nevertheless, one basic background expectation with regard to eating disorders appeared unacceptable for this type of "accommodating" treatment; eventually, the insight of being ill must be maintained, despite feelings of success concerning low body weight or sympathy for pro-ana. If this norm is repeatedly not lived up to, the novice is implicitly refused community membership. This means that the sick role's norms are minimized to the basic norm that the illness must be recognized.

9.7 Difference between online support groups and pro-ana groups

The basic norm of illness recognition, probably points to a desired radical distinction between an online support group on eating disorders and pro-ana groups. The HO threads reveal that pro-ana groups were treated as essentially different from their own community (except for one case in which the difference was scaled down to a low weight competition in pro-ana groups and not in HO). This implies that HO members treat pro-ana sites and groups as "sub-communities of deviants" (Goffman, 1986). Sub-communities of deviants are groups of people who voluntarily and openly accept the social place accorded them, from which they may rebel against certain basic institutions. Willems (2003) argued that groups of social deviants have become increasingly important since the proliferation of new media technology such as the Internet. He claims that the Internet has attracted new forms of deviant behavior, which facilitates identification, but also creates a place to meet and exchange shared "deviant interests." Along this line, pro-ana and pro-mia websites, forums, and so forth can be seen as online communities of deviants. Whether they actually are is a question that goes beyond the scope of this study, but it is important to emphasize that the online support group totally rejects the pro-ana stand. The overarching norm of admitting that one's disordered eating behavior is an illness rather than a lifestyle choice is an implicit distinction from pro-ana groups.

However, some newcomers in the early stages of their illness reveal an attraction to the pro-ana stance and the regulars recognize this. Therefore, we can assume that the rejection of pro-ana is an important step in the early phases of recognizing one's illness. The explicit denunciation of pro-ana continues to work in efforts to convince newcomers that pro-ana is harmful to them. A newcomer who exhibits a pro-ana sympathy is guided along toward the community's norms, rather than scared away from the group. In other words, we cannot judge whether HO and pro-ana are fundamentally different, but the rejection of pro-ana appears to be an important factor in the process of adopting the sick role in the case of eating disorders.

9.8 Conclusion

Sick role theory has proved useful in understanding the initial interactions in an online support group on eating disorders. The early stages of newcomers assuming the sick role are important. Moreover, it needs to be recognized that these stages have recently become even more important, since "falling ill" has become increasingly tied to self-observations rather than professional consultation. Even the medical vocabulary has essentially become disconnected from the medical situation and is used for self-descriptions independent of physicians. I have argued that these changes are related to the communication practices used by online support groups. In the online support group I have analyzed, I discovered clear examples of what the early stages of the sick role truly are. Therefore, the sick role concept requires more recognition for the role of (online, anonymous) peers in the interactions that involve self-observations than was included in the original concept.

We can conclude that the situation involved in entering a forum can be adequately described as the moment that newcomers actually adopt the sick role. A relaxation of normative requirements of the sick role is condoned because it is inherent to the early stages of the sick role. Norm-breaking behavior in terms of feelings of success may actually *confirm* that the newcomer really does have a legitimate reason to join, since this is regarded as typical behavior during the early stages of the illness. Therefore, this stance usually does not jeopardize her/his membership. The interest in accepting more people who are struggling with the illness on their own is given priority over the potential danger of a newcomer's dubious thoughts and attitudes. This means that online communities tolerate stances that are seen as representative of the first stages of the sick role, which includes not yet fulfilling (all) of the normative requirements. At the same time, we must conclude that, even in this situation, however, there is one fundamental norm that must be accepted, and that is the realization that one is ill. This norm is probably what essentially distinguishes the online support group from pro-ana groups.

Chapter 10

Conclusions and discussion

The present study has investigated the first communicative steps of newcomers joining an online support group. It has revealed that socially speaking an online support group is not simply a low threshold service. From an ethnomethodological point of view, it appears that the group was treated as a community and that identity in terms of the illness played an important role in becoming a member of this community. It has been revealed that the communication in an online support forum on eating disorders is characterized by expectations and even normative requirements concerning how to address the forum, how to present yourself and how to describe your problems. The main concern appears to be that newcomers must show that they legitimately wish to join the community. This legitimacy does not only depend on having some experience or acquaintance with the affliction, but moreover on the appropriate attitude towards the disorder. I have analyzed this attitude as a crucial aspect in the process of adopting the sick role.

In the earliest phases of the interactions, nicknames can already begin serving as expressive personal features that conform to what is essential in assuming a legitimate identity in the community (c.f. Thiedeke, 2008: 57-58). Their meanings are closely related to the context in which they are used. In the online support group I analyzed, many nicknames displayed features somehow associated with eating disorders. Moreover, members emphasize that their nicknames are not just labels to sustain anonymity, but represent or constitute an important part of their "selves."

In the actual communication process, various participant types (as categorized by the forum system) seem to behave differently. In the first place, novice members apply interactive strategies to minimize their vulnerability and display legitimacy by using oral discourse features that express ambivalence, or an in-group/expert vocabulary that employs abbreviations and diagnoses. The aim of the first posting seems to be to gain admittance into the community. Acceptance is guaranteed if at least one regular member answers in the affirmative, usually via a formulaic welcome. Hence, a welcome by one member (who can also be a rather recent member her/himself) suffices to include a novice in the group.

If the novice does not display legitimacy in an appropriate manner, however, various regular members will communicate with the newcomer to subtly and kindly urge the novice on in the direction of the "correct" attitude regarding the disorder. (Or, in other cases, the newcomer may not receive any responses at all and communications may be abruptly aborted.) This is how regular members communicate the norms and rules concerning membership in the community.

Finally, moderators play an active role in screening and modifying forum contributions, which can be described as a double role, since they can participate in forum discussions while also assuming the role of censoring certain terms or descriptions from (novice) members' contributions. While novice members do not necessarily adapt to the norms implicitly advocated by regular members, it would be impossible to ignore the moderators' efforts in trying to direct the novices' attitudes. Therefore, the moderators' authority obviously has more influence than that of other, regular members.

I have understood the interactive processes in the online support group as typical for the early stages of the sick role (Parsons, 1951). Online support groups are relatively recent players in the social field of illness. The space they offer in which to discuss illness can be embedded in sick role theory, at least with regard to the early stages of the sick role. However, this only works when the role of peers in the social realm of illness is acknowledged. The role of peers reveals the social dynamics, such as the relevance of the community and identity, which inevitably needs to be taken into account when viewing online support group practices as sick role behavior. A major problem regarding the sick role has been revealed: Newcomers who remain uncertain about their condition are confronted with a choice upon entering an online support group, because they are required to present themselves as ill in order to display legitimacy. However, they may still be ambivalent about presenting themselves as ill, since they either do not yet know whether their symptoms actually fit the diagnosis or they have not yet fully accepted the sick role. In some cases, the other members seem unable or unwilling to deal with the question whether the newcomer is actually ill or not and they leave the question unanswered. In most cases however, they tend to support the newcomer in adopting the sick role. Nevertheless, sometimes they may push a little too hard and scare the newcomer away.

On a methodological level, CA has proved useful for research involving online support groups. It is a valuable alternative to the most frequently used method of "content analysis," which cannot reveal the interactive dynamics in this kind of a group on the level of social action. The present study supports efforts to use CA for the analysis of written communication. The analyses confirm that CA can be applied in a useful manner to naturally occurring, asynchronous CMC data. Despite numerous differences between CMC and spoken interaction, the main premise (viewing language use as social action), as well as certain aspects of sequence organization (i.e., relations between turns such as adjacency pairs) and the use of identities in conversation seem similar for both methods of communication. CMC is still a growing field of communication, and thus, the paths toward analyzing it in the most appropriate ways should be open to further discovery.

The present study has contributed to the increased understanding of the workings of online support groups. The role of legitimacy during the admittance phase seems even more important than has been suggested in earlier research. The social demand for legitimacy works in various directions. It guides newcomers and helps them to accept the illness, which is an important step towards successful treatment and an eventual cure. However, this implicit requirement sometimes also scares them away from the group. At the same time, it also serves to protect regular members, because certain ways of talking about the illness can encourage ill behavior. These findings also point out the fact that despite certain low-threshold features on a structural level (24-hour availability, geographic independence, etc.), entering an online support group is not as unproblematic as it may seem. Social features related to the group as a community and members' identities may actually complicate the low-threshold character of online support groups. The present study therefore leads to the recommendation that a separate sub-forum be added to the HO forum for newcomers who remain unsure about whether they really have an eating disorder. Here, they could pose questions without immediately being included in the community, which would make it easier to avoid the intense levels of insecurity or anxiety felt by some of the newcomers. Meanwhile, other members would not have to be consistently confronted with "intolerable" thoughts about the illness that could actually encourage recidivism regarding eating disorders.

The study revealed that membership norms influence the low threshold character of online support groups. Thus, it would seem unambiguous to assume that the outcomes of the present study can be applied to other types of online support groups. It seems extremely important to understand the ways in which the group treats newcomers, especially when numbers of sub-clinical cases are known to be high. In this sense, the promises of online support activity have not yet been fully exploited. Online support groups have added value to existing health-care services, not only due to anonymity, geographic independence and 24-hour availability, but also because they offer the potential to reach those who do not (manage to) seek help from more institutionalized services. The more knowledge we gain about the actual use of online support groups, the more that these services can ultimately be improved.

Part IV

References and appendix

References

Agha, Asif. (2007). *Language and social relations*. Cambridge: Cambridge University Press.

Alford, Richard. (1988). *Naming and identity: A cross-cultural study of personal naming practices*. New Haven: HRAF Press.

Antaki, Charles, Elisenda Ardévol, Francesc Núnez and Agnès Vayreda. (2005). "For she who knows who she is:" Managing accountability in online forum messages. *Journal of Computer-Mediated Communication, 11* (1), art.6. http://jcmc.indiana.edu/vol11/issue1/antaki.html

Antaki, Charles and Sue Widdicombe. (1998). *Identities in talk*. London: Sage Publications.

Aschenbrenner, Katja. (2001). *Subklinische Essstörungen bei Schülern und Studenten. Epidemiologie, Symptomatik, Prädiktoren für ein gestörtes Essverhalten, anorektische und bulimische Tendenzen*. Unpublished PHD Thesis, Friedrich Schiller University, Jena.

Bassett, Elizabeth and Kathleen O'Riordan. (2002). Ethics of Internet Research: Contesting the Human Subjects Research Model. *Ethics and Information Technology, 4*, 233-249. Retrieved October 21, 2005 from www.nyu.edu/projects/nissenbaum/ethics_bas_full.html

Beauvoir, Simone. (1992/1949). *Das andere Geschlecht; Sitte und Sexus der Frau [Le deuxième sexe]*. Reinbek bei Hamburg: Rowolt Taschenbuch.

Bechar-Israeli, Haya. (1995). From <<Bonehead>> to <<cLoNehEAd>>: Nicknames, play and identity on Internet Relay Chat. *Journal of Computer-Mediated Communication, 1* (2), art.2. http://jcmc.indiana.edu/vol1/issue2/bechar.html

Benwell, Bethan and Elizabeth Stokoe. (2006). *Discourse and identity*. Edinburgh: Edinburgh University Press.

BGBl. I. (2003). *Gesetz zur Regelung des Urheberrechts in der Informationsgesellschaft. 46*, 1774-1788. Retrieved December 4, 2005 from http://www.urheberrecht.org/law/normen/urhg/2003-09-13/text/

Biber, Douglas. (1988). *Variation across speech and writing*. New York: Cambridge University Press.

Biddle, Lucy, Jenny Donovan, Debbie Sharp and David Gunnell. (2007). Explaining non-help-seeking amongst young adults with mental distress: A dynamic interpretive model of illness behaviour. *Sociology of Health and Illness, 29* (7), 983-1002.

Billig, Michael. (1999a). Conversation Analysis and the claims of naivety. *Discourse and society, 10* (4), 572-576.

Billig, Michael. (1999b). Whose terms? Whose ordinariness? Rhetoric and ideology in Conversation Analysis. *Discourse and society, 10* (4), 543-558.

Binik, Yitzchak, James Cantor, Eric Ochs and Marta Meana. (1997). From the couch to the keyboard: Psychotherapy in cyberspace. In S. Kiesler (Ed.), *Culture of the internet* (71-102). Mahwah, New Jersey: Lawrence Erlbaum.

Blaxter, Mildred. (1978). Diagnosis as category and process: The case of alcoholism. *Social Science and Medicine, 12*, 9-17.

Bordo, Susan. (1995). *Unbearable weight: Feminism, western culture and the body*. Berkeley, Los Angeles, London: University of California Press.

Brann, Maria and James Anderson. (2002). E-medicine and health care consumers: Recognizing current problems and possible resolutions for a safer environment. *Health Care Analysis, 10*, 403-415.

Brown, Phil. (1995). Naming and framing: The social construction of diagnosis and illness. *Journal of Health and Social Behavior, 35* (Extra Issue: Forty years of medical sociology: the state of the art and directions for the future), 34-52.

Bruch, Hilde. (2001). *The golden cage: The enigma of anorexia nervosa*. Harvard: University Press.

Buchanan, Elizabeth. (2004). *Readings in virtual research ethics: Issues and controversies*. Hersley, London, Melbourne, Singapore: Information Science Publishing.

Burrows, Roger, Sarah Nettleton, Nicholas Pleace, Brian Loader and Steven Muncer. (2000). Virtual community care? Social policy and the emergence of computer-mediated social support. *Information, Communication and Society, 3* (1), 95-121.

Butler, Judith. (1990). *Gender trouble: Feminism and the subversion of identity.* New York, London: Routledge.

Butler, Judith. (1993). *Bodies that matter: On the discursive limits of sex.* New York, London: Routledge.

Butler, Judith. (1997). *Excitable speech: A politics of the performative.* New York, London: Routledge.

Celio, Angela, Andrew Winzelberg, Parvati Dev and Barr Taylor. (2002). Improving compliance in on-line, structured self-help programs: Evaluation of an eating disorder prevention program. *Journal of Psychiatric Practice, 8* (1), 14-20.

Cherny, Lynn. (1999). *Conversation and community: Chat in a virtual world.* Stanford, CA.: CSLI.

Chesley, E., J. Alberts, J. Klein and R. Kreipe. (2003). Pro or con? Anorexia nervosa and the Internet. *Journal of Adolescent Health, 32* (2), 123-124.

Cohen, Anthony. (1985). *The symbolic construction of community.* London: Routledge.

Conrad, Peter. (1985). The meaning of medications: Another look at compliance. *Social Science and Medicine, 20*, 29-37.

Cooley, Charles. (1909). *Social organization: A study of the larger mind.* New York: Charles Scribner's Sons.

Cotten, Shelia and Sipi Gupta. (2004). Characteristics of online and offline health information seekers and factors that discriminate between them. *Social Science and Medicine, 59* (9), 1795-1806.

Dias, Karen. (2003). The Ana Sanctuary: Women's pro-anorexia narratives in cyberspace. *Journal of International Women's Studies, 4* (2), 31-45. Retrieved May 12, 2005 from http://www.bridgew.us/soas/jiws/April03/Dias.pdf

Döring, Nicola. (1997). Selbsthilfe, Beratung und Therapie im Internet. In B. Batinic (Ed.), *Internet für Psychologen* (421-453). Göttingen, Bern, Toronto, Seattle: Hogrefe.

Döring, Nicola. (2001). Sozialpsychologische Chat-Forschung; Methoden, Theorien, Befunde. In M. Beisswenger (Ed.), *Chat-Kommunikation; Sprache, Interaktion, Sozialität und Identität in synchroner computervermittelter Kommunikation. Perspektiven auf ein interdisziplinäres Forschungsfeld* (141-186). Stuttgard: ibidem Verlag.

Döring, Nicola. (2003). *Sozialpsychologie des Internet; die Bedeutung des Internet für Kommunikationsprozesse, Identitäten, soziale Beziehungen und Gruppen* (2nd ed.). Göttingen, Bern, Toronto, Seattle: Hogrefe.

Drew, Paul. (2005). Conversation Analysis. In K. Fitch and R. Sanders (Eds.), *Handbook of language and social interaction* (71-102). London: Lawrence Erlbaum.

Dubé, Line, Anne Bourhis and Réal Jacob. (2006). Towards a typology of virtual communities of practice. *Interdisciplinary Information, Knowledge, Managment, 1*, 69-93.

Eckert, Penelope and Sally McConnell-Ginet. (1992). Think practically and look locally: Language and gender as community-based practice. *Annual Review Anthropology, 21*, 461-490.

Eckert, Penelope and Sally McConnell-Ginet. (2003). *Language and gender*. Cambridge: University Press Cambridge.

Edwards, Derek. (1997). *Discourse and cognition*. London: Sage Publications.

Edwards, Derek. (1998). The relevant thing about her: Social categories in use. In C. Antaki and S. Widdicombe (Eds.), *Identities in talk* (15-33). London: Sage Publications.

Edwards, Derek and Jonathan Potter. (1992). *Discursive Psychology*. London: Sage Publications.

Edwards, Derek and Elizabeth Stokoe. (2007). Self-help in calls for help with problem neighbours. *Research on language and social interaction, 40* (1), 9-32.

Engel, Antke. (2002). *Wider die Eindeutigkeit; Sexualität und Geschlecht im Fokus queerer Politik der Repräsentation*. Frankfurt/Main: Campus.

Epston, David. (2000). *Separating the person from the problem*. Retrieved February 15, 2007, from www.narrativeapproaches.com/antianorexia%20folder/anti_anorexia_index.htm

Erikson, Erik. (1968). *Identity, youth and crisis*. New York: W.W. Norton.

Ess, Charles and Association of Internet Research AoIR. (2002). *Ethical decision-making and Internet research; recommendations from the aoir ethics working committee*. Retrieved October 21, 2005 from www.aoir.org/reports/ethics.pdf

Farrell, Em. (1995). *Lost for words: The psychoanalysis of Anorexia and Bulimia*. New York: Other Press.

Favaro, A. and P. Santonastaso. (1997). Suicidality in eating disorders: Clinical and psychological correlates. *Acta Psychiatr Scand, 95*, 508-514.

Finn, Jerry. (1999). An exploration of helping processes in an online self-help group focussing on issues of disabilities. *Health and Social Work, 24*, 220-231.

Fitzgerald, Richard and William Housley. (2002). Identity, categorization and sequential organization: The sequential and categorial flow of identity in a radio phone-in. *Discourse and Society, 13* (5), 579-602.

Fornari, Victor, Myra Kaplan, David Sandberg, Michael Matthews, Neil Skolnick and Jack Katz. (1992). Depressive and anxiety disorders in anorexia nervosa and bulimia nervosa. *International Journal of Eating Disorders, 12* (1), 21-29.

Foucault, Michel. (1967). *Madness and civilization*. UK: Tavistock Publications.

Foucault, Michel. (1972). *The archeology of knowledge and the discourse on language*. New York: Pantheon.

Foucault, Michel. (1977). *Discipline and punish: The birth of the prison*. New York: Random House.

Foucault, Michel. (1986). *The care of the self: The history of sexuality* (Vol. 3). New York: Vintage.

Fox, Nick, Katie Ward and Alan O'Rourke. (2005). Pro-anorexia, weight-loss drugs and the internet: An "anti-recovery" explanatory model of anorexia. *Sociology of Health and Illness, 27* (7), 944-971.

Francis, David and Stephen Hester. (2004). *An invitation to ethnomethodology: Language, society and interaction*. London: Sage Publications.

Frank, Arthur. (1994). Reclaiming an orphan genre: The first-person narrative of illness. *Literature and Medicine, 13* (1), 1-21.

Friedan, Betty. (1966/1963). *Der Weiblichkeitswahn oder die Mystifizierung der Frau [The feminine mystique]*. Reinbek bei Hamburg: Rowohlt Verlag.

Galegher, Jolene, Lee Sproull and Sara Kiesler. (1998). Legitimacy, authority and community in electronic support groups. *Written Communication, 15* (4), 493-530.

Garfinkel, Harold. (1967). *Studies in ethnomethodology*. Englewood Cliffs N.J.: Prentice-Hall.

Gerhards, Jürgen. (2003). *Die Moderne und ihre Vornamen: eine Einladung in die Kultursoziologie*. Opladen and Wiesbaden: Westdeutscher Verlag.

Gerhardt, Uta. (1989). *Ideas about illness: An intellectual and political history of medical sociology*. London: Macmillan.

Gerlinghoff, Monica and Herbert Backmund. (2004). Essstörungen im Kindes- und Jugendalter; Anorexia norvosa, Bulimia nervosa, Binge Eating Disorder. *Bundesgesundheitsbl. – Gesundheitsforsch. – Gesundheitsschutz, 47*, 246-250.

Giddens, Anthony. (1984). *The constitution of society: Outline of the theory of structuration*. Cambridge: Polity Press.

Goffman, Erving. (1956). The nature of deference and demeanor. *American Anthropologist, 58*, 473-502.

Goffman, Erving. (1959). *The presentation of the self in everyday life*. Harmondsworth: Penguin.

Goffman, Erving. (1961). *Asylums: Essays on the social situation of mental patients and other inmates.* New York: Doubleday Anchor Books.

Goffman, Erving. (1967). *Interaction ritual: Essays on face-to-face behavior*. Garden City, New York: Doubleday Anchor Books.

Goffman, Erving. (1974). *Frame analysis: An essay on the organization of experience*. New York: Harper.

Goffman, Erving. (1982/1971). *Das Individuum im öffentlichem Austausch [Relations in public: microstudies of the public order]*. Frankfurt/Main: Suhrkamp.

Goffman, Erving. (1986). *Stigma; notes on the management of spoiled identity*. New York: Siman and Schuster Inc.

Goldner, Elliot, Laird Birmingham and Victoria Smye. (1997). Addressing treatment refusal in Anorexia Nervosa; clinical, ethical and legal considerations. In D. Garner and P. Garfinkel (Eds.), *Handbook of treatment for eating disorders* (2nd ed., 450-461). New York: Guilford Press.

Grosz, Elizabeth. (1994). *Volatile Bodies*. Bloomington: Indiana University Press.

Grunfeld, Robert, Masood Zangeneh and Alex Grunfeld. (2004). Stigmatization dialogue: deconstruction and content analysis. *International Journal of Mental Health and Addiction, 1* (2), 1-14.

Gugutzer, Robert. (2005). Der Körper als Identitätsmedium: Eßstörungen. In M. Schroer (Ed.), *Soziologie des Körpers* (323-355). Frankfurt/Main: Suhrkamp.

Habermas, Tillman. (1990). *Heißhunger. Historische Bedingungender Bulimia nervosa*. Frankfurt/Main: Fischer.

Habermas, Tillman. (1992). Possible effects of the medical classification of bulimia nervosa. *British Journal of Medical Psychology, 65*, 317-334.

Habermas, Tillman. (2000). "Liegt's wirklich an der Werbung? " Soziokulturelle Determinanten moderner Essstörungen. In M. Gastpar, H. Remschmidt and W. Senf (Eds.), *Essstörungen. Neue Erkenntnisse und Forschungsperspektiven* (11-28). Berlin: Wissenschaft und Praxis.

Hacohen, Gonen. (2007). *Local practices of local identities: Callers' types in Israel radio phone-in programs*. Paper presented at the 10th International Pragmatics Conference, Göteborg, Sweden.

Hahn, Alois. (2003). Aufmerksamkeit und Normalität. In J. Link, T. Loer and H. Neuendorff (Eds.), *"Normalität" im Diskursnetz soziologischer Begriffe* (23-37). Heidelberg: Synchron.

Hall, Stuart. (1997). The work of representation . In S. Hall (Ed.), *Representation. Cultural representations and signifying practices.* (15-71). London: Sage Publications.

Hall, Stuart. (2004). Who needs identity? In P. d. Gay, J. Evans and P. Redman (Eds.), *Identity: A reader* (15-30). London: Sage Publications.

Hellinger, Marlis and Hadumod Bußmann. (2001). *Gender across languages; the linguistic representation of women and men.* Amsterdam and Philadelphia: John Benjamins Publishing Company.

Hepworth, Julie. (1999). *The social construction of anorexia nervosa.* London: Sage Publications.

Heritage, John. (1984). *Garfinkel and ethnomethodology.* Cambridge: Polity Press.

Heritage, John. (2001). Goffman, Garfinkel and Conversation Analysis. In M. Wetherell, S. Taylor and S. J. Yates (Eds.), *Discourse theory and practice* (47-56). London: Sage Publications.

Heritage, John and Jeffrey Robinson. (2006). Accounting for the visit: Giving reasons for seeking medical care. In J. Heritage and D. Maynard (Eds.), *Communication in medical care: Interaction between primary care physicians and patients* (48-85). New York: Cambridge University Press.

Herring, Susan. (1996). Linguistic and critical analysis of Computer-Mediated Communication; Some ethical and scholarly considerations. *The Information Society, 12* (2), 153-168.

Herring, Susan. (1999). Interactional coherence in CMC. *Journal of Computer-Mediated Communication, 4* (4) http://jcmc.indiana.edu/vol4/issues4/herring.html

Herring, Susan. (2001). Computer-Mediated Discourse. In D. Schiffrin (Ed.), *The handbook of discourse analysis* (612-634). Malden, Mass.: Blackwell.

Herring, Susan. (2004). Computer-Mediated Discourse Analysis: An approach to researching online behavior. In S. Barab, R. Kling and J. Gray (Eds.), *Designing for virtual communities in the service of learning* (338-376). New York: Cambridge University Press.

Herring, Susan. (2008 in press). Virtual community. In L. M. Given (Ed.), *Encyclopedia of qualitative research methods*. Thousand Oaks: Sage Publications.

Herzlich, Claudine and Janine Pierret. (1985). The social construction of the patient: Patients and illnesses in other ages. *Social Science and Medicine, 20* (2), 145-151.

Herzog, Wolfgang, Dietrich Munz and Horst Kächele. (2004). *Essstörungen: Therapieführer und psychodynamische Behundlungskonzepte*. Stuttgart: Schattauer.

Höflich, Joachim. (1996). *Technisch vermittelte interpersonale Kommunikation*. Opladen and Wiesbaden: Westdeutscher Verlag.

Hohmeier, Jürgen. (1975). Stigmatisierung als sozialer Definitionsprozess. In M. Busten and J. Hohmeier (Eds.), *Stigmatisierung* (55-124). Neuwied: Luchterhand Verlag.

Hopper, Robert. (1992). *Telephone conversation*. Bloomington: Indiana University Press.

Houtkoop, Hanneke and Tom Koole. (2000). *Taal in actie: Hoe mensen communiceren met taal*. Bussum: Coutinho.

Hutchby, Ian. (2000). *Conversation and technology: From the telephone to the internet*. Cambridge: Polity Press.

Hutchby, Ian and Robin Wooffitt. (1998). *Conversation Analysis: Principles, practices and applications*. Cambridge: Polity Press.

Jacobson, David. (1999). Impression formation in cyberspace: Online expectations and offline experiences in text-based virtual communities. *Journal of Computer-Mediated Communication, 5* (1) http://jcmc.indiana.edu/vol5/issue1/jacobson.html

Jahandarie, Khosrow. (1999). *Spoken and written discourse: A multidisciplinary perspective*. Stamford, Connecticut: Ablex Publishing Company.

Jaworski, Adam and Nikolas Coupland. (1999). *The discourse reader*. London: Routledge.

Johnson, Jan-Are, Jan Rosenvinge and Deede Gammon. (2002). Online group interaction and mental health: An analysis of three online discussion forums. *Scandinavian Journal of Psychology, 43*, 445-449.

Karwauts, Andreas. (1997). *Eßstörungen*. Retrieved 10.03.06, 2007, from http://www.wien.gv.at/who/gb/97/index.htm

Keel, Pamela and Kelly Klump. (2003). Are eating disorders culture-bound syndromes? Implications for conceptualizing their etiology. *Psychological Bulletin, 129* (5), 747-769.

Kennedy, Helen. (2006). Beyond anonymity, or future directions for internet identity research. *New Media and Society, 8* (6), 859-876.

Kiesler, Sara, Jane Siegel and Timothy McGuire. (1984). Social psychological aspects of computer-mediated communication. *American Psychologist, 39* (10), 1123-1134.

King, Storm. (1994). Analysis of electronic support groups for recovering addicts. *Interpersonal Computing and Technology: An Electronic Journal for the 21st Century, 2* (3), 47-56. Retrieved November 13, 2006 from http://webpages.charter.net/stormking/elect.html

King, Storm. (1996). Researching Internet communities: Proposed ethical guidelines for the reporting of the results. *The Information Society, 12* (2), 119-127.

Konishi, Toshiko. (1991). *Language and thought: A cross-cultural study on the connotations of gender.* Unpublished PhD Thesis, University of California, Los Angeles.

Koole, Tom. (1997). The role of ethnography in the analysis of institutional discourse. In L. Lentz and H. P. Maat (Eds.), *Discourse analysis and evaluation* (59-86). Amsterdam: Rodopi.

Korenman, Joan and Nancy Wyatt. (1996). Group dynamics in an e-mail forum. In S. Herring (Ed.), *Computer-Mediated Communication: Linguistic, social and cross-cultural perspectives* (225-242). Amsterdam and Philadelphia: John Benjamins Publishing Company.

Kral, G. and C. Presslich. (2002). Analyse und Evaluation von Selbsthilfe-Ressourcen im Internet (www) anhand eines Forums für Menschen mit Essstörungen. In M. Brüstle (Ed.), *Kommunikation der Zukunft – Zukunft der Kommunikation* (53-63). Bonn: Deutscher Psychologenverlag.

Lamerichs, Joyce. (2003). *Discourse of Support: Exploring online discussions on depression.* Unpublished PHD Thesis, Wageningen University, Netherlands, Wageningen.

Lamerichs, Joyce and Hedwig Te Molder. (2003). Computer-Mediated Communication: From a cognitive to a discursive model. *New Media and Society, 5* (4), 451-473.

Lasker, Judith, Ellen Sogolow and Rebecca Sharim. (2005). The role of an online community for people with a rare disease: Content analysis of messages posted on a primary biliary cirrhosis mailinglist. *Journal of Medical Internet Research, 7* (1), e10. Retrieved April 7, 2008 from http://www.jmir.org/2005/1/e10

Lave, Jean and Etienne Wenger. (1991). *Situated learning: Legitimate peripheral participation*. Cambridge: Cambridge University Press.

Lawson, Danielle. (2004). Blurring the boundaries: Ethical considerations for online research using synchronous CMC forums. In E. A. Buchanan (Ed.), *Readings in virtual research ethic: Issues and controversies* (80-100). Hersley, London, Melbourne, Singapore: Information Science Publishing.

Lea, Martin, Tim O'Shea, Pat Fung and Russell Spears. (1992). "Flaming" in computer-mediated communication: Observations, explanations, implications. In M. Lea (Ed.), *Contexts of computer-mediated communication* (89-112). New York: Harvester Wheatsheaf.

Leiberich, Peter. (2005, December 23). *Die Hungrig-Online Umfrage 2003: wichtigste Ergebnisse des Hungrig-Online NutzerInnen-Umfrage aus dem Jahr 2003*. Retrieved August 22, 2007, from http://www.hungrig-online.de/forum/ubbthreads.php/ubb/showflat/Number/80608#Post80608

Leiberich, Peter, Jan Nedoschill, Marius Nickel, Thomas Loew and Karin Tritt. (2004). Selbsthilfe und Beratung im Internet: mündige Benutzer können die Arzt-Patienten-Beziehung neu gestalten. *Medizinische Klinik, 99* (5), 263-268.

Lester, Rebecca. (1997). The (dis)embodied self in anorexia nervosa. *Social Science Medicine, 44* (4), 479-489.

Liebsch, Katharina. (2007, May 2.). *Passung und Anpassung; körperpolitische Überlegungen zum Zusammenhang von Geschlecht und Zugehörigkeit.* Paper presented at the CGC-Interdisciplinary Colloquium "Belonging and Participation," Frankfurt/Main.

Link, Jürgen. (1999). *Versuch über den Normalismus; wie Normalität produziert wird* (2nd. ed.). Opladen and Wiesbaden: Westdeutscher Verlag.

Loader, Brian, Steve Muncer, Roger Burrows, Nicolas Pleace and Sarah Nettleton. (2002). Medicine on the line? Computer-mediated support and advice for people with diabetes. *International Journal of Social Welfare, 11*, 53-65.

Lock, Andrew, David Epston and Richard Maisel. (2004). Countering that which is called anorexia. *Narrative Inquiry, 14* (2), 275-301.

Lorenz, Konrad. (1943). Die angeborenen Formen möglicher Erfahrung. *Zeitschrift für Tierpsychologie, 5* (2), 235-409.

Luhmann, Niklas. (1990). Der medizinische Code. In N. Luhmann (Ed.), *Soziologische Aufklärung* (Vol. 5, 183-195). Opladen and Wiesbaden: Westdeutscher Verlag.

Lyons, Elizabeth, Matthias Mehl and James Pennebaker. (2006). Pro-anorexics and recovering anorexics differ in their linguistic internet self-presentation. *Journal of Psychosomatic Research, 60*, 253-256.

Lyons, John. (1995). *Linguistic semantics: An introduction*. Cambridge: Cambridge University Press.

Malson, Helen. (1998). *The Thin Woman: Feminism, post-structuralism and the social psychology of anorexia nervosa*. London and New York: Routledge.

McKay, Susan. (2001). Beyond biomedicine: Renegotiating the sick role for postmodern conditions. *Journal of Media and Culture, 4* (3). Retrieved May 4, 2008 from http://journal.media-culture.org.au/0106/bio.php

Mechanic, David. (1978). *Medical Sociology* (2 ed.). New York: Free Press.

Meehan, Andrew. (1989). Assessing the "police-worthiness" of citizen's complaints to the police: Accountability and the negotiation of "facts." In D. T. Helm, W. T. Anderson, A. J. Meehan and A. W. Rawls (Eds.), *The interactional order: New directions in the study of social order* (116-140). New York: Irvington.

Millett, Kate. (1985/1969). *Sexus und Herrschaft: die Tyrannei des Mannes in unserer Gesellschaft [Sexual politics]*. Reinbek bei Hamburg: Rowohlt Verlag.

Mills, Sara. (2004). *Discourse Analysis* (2nd ed.). London: Routledge.

Misoch, Sabina. (2004). *Identitäten im Internet: Selbstdarstellung auf privaten Homepages*. Konstanz: UVK.

Münsterman, Sandra and Gisela Steins. (2003). Stigmatisierung essgestörter Frauen in Abhängigkeit vom diagnostischen Ansatz und der Form der Essstörung. *Zeitschrift für Klinische Psychologie und Psychotherapie, 32* (1), 1-9.

Nettleton, Sarah, Ian Watt, Lisa O'Malley and Philip Duffey. (2005). Understanding the narratives of people who live with medically unexplained illness. *Patient Education and Counselling, 56* (2), 205-210.

Norris, Mark, Katherine Boydell, Leora Pinhas and Debra Katzman. (2006). Ana and the internet; a review of Pro-Anorexia Websites. *International Journal of Eating Disorders, 39* (6), 443-447.

O'Brian, Karina and Nora Vincent. (2003). Psychiatric comorbidity in anorexia and bulimia nervosa: Nature, prevalence and causal relationships. *Clinical Psychology Review, 23*, 57-74.

Oelkers, Susanne. (2004). Warum Adam und Eva? Vornamengebung und Geschlecht. In K. M. Eichhoffcyrus (Ed.), *Adam, Eva und die Sprache* (Vol. 5, 133-147). Mannheim, Leipzig, Wien, Zürich: Dudenverlag.

Olson, Greta. (2003). *Reading eating disorders: Writings on bulimia and anorexia as confessions of American culture*. Frankfurt/Main: Lang.

Opielka, Michael. (2004). *Gemeinschaft in Gesellschaft; soziologie nach Hegel und Parsons*. Wiesbaden: VS Verlag.

Orbach, Susie. (2001). *Hunger strike: Starving amidst plenty*. New York: Other Press.

Paccagnella, Luciano. (1997). Getting the seat of your pants dirty: Strategies for ethnographic research on virtual communities. *Journal of Computer-Mediated Communication, 3* (1), art. 4. http://jcmc.indiana.edu/vol3/issue1/paccagnella.html

Panyametheekul, Siriporn and Susan Herring. (2003). Gender and turn allocation in a Thai chat room. *Journal of Computer-Mediated Communication, 9* (1) http://jcmc.indiana.edu/vol9/issue1/panya_herring.html

Parsons, Talcott. (1939). The professions and social structure. *Social Forces, 17*, 457-467.

Parsons, Talcott. (1951). *The social system*. London: Tavistock.

Pomerantz, Anita. (1984). Agreeing and disagreeing with assessments: some features of preferred/dispreferred turn shapes. In J. M. Atkinson and J. Heritage (Eds.), *Structures of social action: Studies in Conversation Analysis* (57-101). Cambridge: Cambridge University Press.

Pomerantz, Anita. (1986). Extreme case formulations. *Human Studies, 9*, 219-229.

Potter, Jonathan. (1996). *Representing reality: Discourse, rhetoric and social construction*. London: Sage Publications.

Potter, Jonathan and Margaret Wetherell. (1987). *Discourse and Social Psychology: Beyond attitudes and behaviour*. London: Sage Publications.

Preece, Jenny. (2000). *Online communities: Designing, usability and supporting sociability*. UK: Wiley.

Preece, Jenny, Blair Nonnecke and Dorine Andrews. (2004). The top 5 reasons for lurking: Improving community experiences for everyone. *Computers in Human Behavior, 2* (2), 201-223.

Radley, Alan and Michael Billig. (1996). Accounts of health and illness: Dilemmas and representations. *Sociology of Health and Illness, 18* (2), 220-240.

Rains, Stephen. (2008). Health at high speed: Broadband internet access, health communication, and the digital divide. *Communication Research, 35* (3), 283-297.

Reindl, Sheila. (2001). *Sensing the self: Women's recovery from bulimia*. Cambridge Mass. and London: Harvard University Press.

Rheingold, Howard. (2000). *The virtual community. Homesteading on the Electronic Frontier* (2nd ed.). Cambridge: MIT Press.

Rich, Emma. (2006). Anorexic dis(connection): Managing anorexia as an illness and an identity. *Sociology of Health and Illness, 28* (3), 284-305.

Rintal, Sean, Joan Mulholland and Jeffrey Pittam. (2001). First things first: Internet relay chat openings. *Journal of Computer-Mediated Communication, 6* (3) http://jcmc.indiana.edu/vol6/issue3/rintel.html

Rymes, Betsy. (1996). Naming as social practice: The case of Little Creeper from Diamond Street. *Language and Society, 25* (2), 237-260.

Sacks, Harvey. (1972). An initial investigation of the usability of conversational data for doing sociology. In D. Sudnow (Ed.), *Studies in social interaction* (31-74). Glencoe, I.L.: Free Press.

Sacks, Harvey. (1974). An analysis of the course of a joke's telling in conversation. In J. Sherzer and D. Baumann (Eds.), *Explorations in the ethnography of communication* (337-353). Cambridge: Cambridge University Press.

Sacks, Harvey. (1984). Notes on methodology. In J. M. Atkinson and J. Heritage (Eds.), *Structures of social action; studies in Conversation Analysis* (21-27). Cambridge: Cambridge University Press.

Sacks, Harvey. (1992). *Lectures on conversation* (Vol. 1,2). Oxford: Blackwell.

Sandaunet, Anne-Grete. (2008). The challenge of fitting in: Non-participation and withdrawal from an online self-help group for breast cancer patients. *Sociology of Health, 30* (1), 131-144.

Schegloff, Emanuel. (1968). Sequencing in conversational openings. *American Anthropologist, 70* (6), 1075-1095.

Schegloff, Emanuel. (1979). Identification and recognition in telephone conversation openings. In G. Psathas (Ed.), *Everyday language: Studies in ethnomethodology*. New York: Ervington.

Schegloff, Emanuel. (1984). On some questions and ambiguities in conversations. In J. M. Atkinson and J. Heritage (Eds.), *Structures of social interaction* (266-298). Cambridge: Cambridge University Press.

Schegloff, Emanuel. (1986). The routine as achievement. *Human Studies, 9*, 111-151.

Schegloff, Emanuel. (1992). Repair after next turn: The last structurally provided for place for the defense of intersubjectivity in conversation. *American Journal of Sociology, 95* (5), 1295-1345.

Schegloff, Emanuel. (1997). Whose text? Whose context? *Discourse and society, 8* (2), 165-187.

Schegloff, Emanuel. (1999a). Naivety vs sophistication or discipline vs self-indulgence: A rejoinder to Billig. *Discourse and society, 10* (4), 577-582.

Schegloff, Emanuel. (1999b). Schegloff's texts as "Billig's data:" A critical reply. *Discourse and society, 10* (4), 558-572.

Schegloff, Emanuel. (2007). A tutorial on membership categorization. *Journal of Pragmatics, 39*, 462-482.

Schegloff, Emanuel and Harvey Sacks. (1973). Opening up closings. *Semiotica, 8* (4), 289-327.

Schoemaker, Casper. (2002). *Anorexia bestaat niet: Het beeld van anorexia nervosa in de media*. Amsterdam: Archipel.

Schultz, P.N. (2002). Providing information to patients with a rare cancer: Using internet discussion forums to address the needs of patients with medullary thryoid carcinoma. *Clinical Journal of Oncology Nursing, 6*, 219-222.

Scott, Marvin and Stanford Lyman. (1968). Accounts. *Americal Sociological Review, 33* (1), 46-62.

Segall, Alexander. (1976). The sick role concept: Understanding social behavior. *Journal of Health and Social Behavior, 17* (2), 163-170.

Shisslak, Catherine, Marjorie Crago and Linda Estes. (1995). The spectrum of eating disturbances. *International Journal of Eating Disorders, 18* (3), 209-219.

Shuman, Amy. (1986). *Storytelling rights: The uses of oral and written texts by urban adolescents*. Cambridge: Cambridge University Press.

Sixsmith, Judith and Craig D. Murray. (2001). Ethical issues in the documentary data analysis of Internet posts and archives. *Qualitative-Health-Research, 11* (3), 423-432.

Smith, Dorothy. (1978). K is mentally ill: The anatomy of a factual account. *Sociology, 12*, 23-53.

Smith, Marc and Peter Kollock. (1999). *Communities in cyberspace*. London: Routledge.

Smyres, Kerrie M. (1999). Virtual corporeality: Adolescent girls and their bodies in cyberspace. *Research Methodology Online, 6*. Retrieved February 13, 2006 from www.cybesociety.com/files/6_3_girlsandbodiesonline.html

Speer, Susan A. and Jonathan Potter. (2002). From performatives to practices; Judith Butler, discursive psychology and the management of heterosexist talk. In P. McIlvenny (Ed.), *Talking gender and sexuality* (151-180). Amsterdam and Philadelphia: John Benjamins Company.

Stegbauer, Christian. (2000). Begrenzungen und Strukturen internetbasierter Kommunikationsgruppen. In C. Thimm (Ed.), *Soziales im Netz: Sprache, Beziehungen und Kommunikationskulturen im Internet* (18-38). Opladen and Wiesbaden: Westdeutscher Verlag.

Stommel, Wyke. (2007). "Mein Nick bin ich!" Nicknames in a German forum on eating disorders. *Journal of Computer-Mediated Communication, 13* (1), art. 8. http://jcmc.indiana.edu/vol13/issue1/stommel.html

Stommel, Wyke. (2008). Conversation Analysis and Community of Practice: An approach to studying online community. In J. Androutsopoulos and M. Beißwenger (Eds.), *Data and methods in computer-mediated discourse analysis*. Special Issue: Language@internet, art.5. http://www.languageatinternet.de/articles/2008

Subrahmanyam, Kaveri, Patricia M. Greenfield and Brendesha Tynes. (2004). Constructing sexuality and identity in an online teen chat room. *Journal of Applied Developmental Psychology, 25* (6), 651-666.

Suchman, Edward. (1965). Stages of illness and medical care. *Journal of Health and Human Behavior, 6*, 114-128.

Sundèn, Jenny. (2003). *Material virtualities: Approaching online textual embodiment*. New York: Lang.

Tajfel, Henry. (1982). *Social identity and intergroup relations*. Cambridge: Cambridge University Press.

Tajfel, Henry and Jonathan Turner. (1986). The Social Identity Theory of intergroup behaviour. In S. Worchel and W. G. Austin (Eds.), *Psychology of intergroup relations* (7-24). Chicago: Nelson-Hall.

Tan, Jacinta, Tony Hope and Anne Stewart. (2003). Anorexia Nervosa and personal identity: The accounts of patients and their parents. *International Journal of Law and Psychiatry, 26* (5), 533-548.

Ten Have, Paul. (1999). *Doing Conversation Analysis: A practical guide*. London: Sage Publications.

Thiedeke, Udo. (2008). Die Gemeinschaften der Eigensinnigen: Interaktionsmediale Kommunikationsbedingungen und virtuelle Gemeinschaften. In F. von Gross, W. Marotzki and U. Sander (Eds.), *Internet – Bildung – Gemeinschaft* (45-71). Wiesbaden: VS Verlag.

Thiedeke, Udo (Ed.). (2000). *Virtuelle Gruppen: Charakteristika und Problemdimensionen*. Opladen and Wiesbaden: Westdeutscher Verlag.

Thimm, Caja and Heidi Ehmer. (2000). "Wie im richtigen Leben...:" soziale Identität und sprachliche Kommunikation in einer Newsgroup. In C. Thimm (Ed.), *Soziales im Netz; Sprache, Beziehungen und Kommunikationskulturen im Internet* (220-239). Opladen and Wiesbaden: Westdeutscher Verlag.

Tracy, Karin. (2002). *Everyday talk: Building and reflecting identities*. New York: Guilford Press.

Treasure, Janet, Ulrike Schmidt and Eric van Furth. (2005). *The essential handbook of eating disorders*. Southern Gate, Chichester, UK: John Wiley and Sons.

Turkle, Sherry. (1995). Life on the screen: Identity in the age of the internet. New York: Simon and Schuster.

Van Hoeken, Daphne, Jacob Seidell and Hans Wijbrand Hoek. (2005). Epidemiology. In J. Treasure, U. Schmidt and E. Van Furth (Eds.), *The essential handbook of eating disorders* (11-34). Southern Gate, Chichester: John Wiley and Sons.

Vandereycken, Walter, Ron van Deth and Rolf Meerman. (2003). *Wundermädchen, Hungerkünstler, Magersucht: eine Kulturgeschichte zu Essstörungen*. Weinheim, Basel, Berlin: Betlz.

Waldvogel, Joan. (2007). Greetings and closings in workplace email. *Journal of Computer-Mediated Communication, 12* (2), art. 6. http://jcmc.indiana.edu/vol12/issue2/waldvogel.html

Walstrom, Mary. (2000a). "The eating disorder is not you." Applying Bakhtin's theories in analyzing narrative co-construction in an internet support group. *Studies in Symbolic Interaction, 23*, 241-260.

Walstrom, Mary. (2000b). "You know who is the thinnest?" Combating surveillance and creating safety in coping with eating disorders online. *CyberPsychology and Behavior, 3* (5), 761-783.

Waskul, Dennis and Mark Douglas. (1996). Considering the electronic participant: Some polemical observations on the ethics of on-line research. *The Information Society, 12*, 129-139.

Weeks, Peter. (1995). The microsociology of everyday life. In S. Hale (Ed.), *Controversies in sociology* (449-472). Toronto: Copp Clark.

Wellman, Barry. (1988). *Social structures: A network approach*. Cambridge: Cambridge University Press.

Wellman, Barry. (1997). An electronic group is virtually a social network. In S. Kiesler (Ed.), *Culture of the internet* (179-208). Mahwah, New Jersey: Lawrence Erlbaum.

Wenger, Etienne. (2004). *Communities of Practice: Learning, meaning and identity*. Cambridge: Cambridge University Press.

West, Candace and Don H. Zimmerman. (1987). Doing Gender. *Gender and society, 1* (2), 125-151.

Westenhöfer, Joachim. (2001). Prevalence of eating disorders and weight control practices in Germany in 1990 and 1997. *International Journal of Eating Disorders, 29*, 477-481.

Wetherell, Margaret. (1998). Positioning and interpretive repertoires: Conversation Analysis and Post-structuralism in dialogue. *Discourse and society, 9* (3), 387-412.

Whalen, Marilyn and Don Zimmerman. (1990). Describing trouble: Practical epistemology in citizen calls to the police. *Language in Society, 19*, 465-492.

Widdicombe, Sue and Robin Wooffitt. (1995). *The language of youth subcultures: Social identity in action*. Hemel Hempstead: Harvester Wheatsheaf.

Wilkinson, Sue and Celia Kitzinger. (2007). Conversation Analysis, gender and sexuality. In A. Weatherall, B. Watson and C. Gallois (Eds.),

Language, Discourse and Social Psychology (207-230). London: Palgrave/Macmillan.

Willems, Herbert. (2003). Normalität, Normalisierung, Normalismus. In J. Link, T. Loer and H. Neuendorff (Eds.), *"Normalität" im Diskursnetz soziologischer Begriffe* (51-84). Heidelberg: Synchron.

Williams, Gareth. (1989). "Hope for the humblest? " The role of self help in chronic illness: The case of anklosing spondyliitis. *Sociology of Health and Illness, 11* (2), 135-159.

Wilson, Thomas. (1971). Normative and interpretive paradigms in sociology. In J. Douglas (Ed.), *Understanding everyday life: Toward the reconstruction of sociological knowledge* (57-79). London: Routledge and Kegan Paul.

Winzelberg, Andrew. (1997). The analysis of an electronic support group for individuals with eating disorders. *Computers in Human Behavior, 13* (3), 393-407.

Wirtz, Mica. (2008). Die Magie der Zahlen: Überlegungen zum aktuellen Diskurs um Übergewicht und Adipositas. In C. Camus, A. Hornung, F. Imlinger, A. Kolbe, M. Noll and I. Stauffer (Eds.), *Im Zeichen des Geschlechts: Repräsentationen, Konstruktionen, Interventionen.* Königstein/Taunus: Helmer Verlag.

Wooffitt, Robin. (1992). Telling tales of the unexpected: The organization of factual discourse. Savage, Maryland: Barns and Noble Books.

Yates, Simeon J. (1996). Oral and written linguistic aspects of computer-conferencing. In S. Herring (Ed.), *Computer-mediated communication: Linguistic, social and crosscultural perspectives* (29-46). Amsterdam and Philadelphia: John Benjamins Company.

Yates, Simeon J. (1997). Gender, identity and CMC. *Journal of Computer Assisted Learning, 13*, 281-290.

Zelenkauskaite, A. and Susan Herring. (2006). Gender encoding of typographical elements in Lithuanian and Croatian IRC. In F. Sudweeks and C. Ess (Eds.), *Proceedings of Cultural Attitudes Towards Technology and Culture 2006 (CATaC'06).* Murdoch, Australia: Murdoch University Press. Preprint, retrieved June 11, 2008: http://ella.slis.indiana.edu/~herring/catac2006.pdf.

Zimmerman, Don. (1998). Identity, context and interaction. In C. Antaki and S. Widdicombe (Eds.), *Identities in talk* (87-106). London: Sage Publications.

Appendix

Email to HO-members and HO-moderators with request for publication of thread excerpts:

Liebe (ehemalige) HO-Moderatorin, lieber (ehemaliger) HO-Moderator, ODER
Liebe (ehemalige) HO-Userin, lieber (ehemaliger) HO-User,

mein Name ist Wyke Stommel. Im Rahmen meiner Promotion an der Universität Frankfurt untersuche ich **Beiträge im Hungrig-Online-Forum aus dem Jahr 2005 und früher**. Es geht mir dabei um die Frage, wie Identität(en) und Gemeinschaft(sbildung) in den Threads konstruiert werden. Die Untersuchung ist interdisziplinär, denn sie stützt sich auf sowohl linguistische als auch soziologische/sozialpsychologische Theorien.

Hiermit bitte ich Sie um die Zustimmung für die Veröffentlichung eines kleinen Ausschnittes Ihrer Beiträge in Hungrig-Online-Forum im Rahmen meiner Forschungsarbeit.

Es handelt sich dabei um den folgenden Ausschnitt:
[…]

Ich versichere, dass ich aus rechtlichen und ethischen Gründen alle aus dem Hungrig-Online-Forum erhobenen Daten und Informationen **vollständig anonymisieren** werde. Eventuell enthaltene personenbezogene Daten werden gelöscht oder so verändert, dass kein Rückschluss auf Ihre Identität mehr möglich ist. Der Verein Hungrig-Online e.V. befürwortet und unterstützt nach genauer Prüfung und unter der oben genannten Bedingung mein Forschungsvorhaben zur Untersuchung von ausgewählten Beiträgen aus dem öffentlichen Forum.

Falls Sie mir Ihre Zustimmung zur Veröffentlichung kurzer Ausschnitten aus ihren Beiträgen nicht geben möchten, dann bitte ich Sie ebenfalls, mir eine **Ablehnung per E-Mail** zu schicken: Stommel@soz.uni-frankfurt.de. Ich werde Ihre Beiträge dann ausdrücklich aus der Untersuchung ausnehmen.

Falls Sie nicht auf meine E-Mail reagieren, werde ich so vorgehen, als ob kein ausdrücklicher Widerspruch vorliegt. Gegebenenfalls werde ich dann kleine Ausschnitte einzelner Beiträge, die garantiert anonymisiert sind, veröffentlichen.

Für weitere Fragen können Sie sich direkt an mich oder auch an Herrn Dr.-Ing. Wolfgang Gawlik, ehemaliger Vorstandsmitglied des Vereins Hungrig-Online e.V. (wolfgang.gawlik@hungrig-online.de), wenden.

Ich bedanke mich schon im Voraus bei Ihnen. Ausschnitte und Ergebnisse meiner Dissertation werde ich sicher bei Hungrig-Online präsentieren.

Mit freundlichen Gruß,

Wyke Stommel

Wyke Stommel c/o Cornelia Goethe Centrum
Johann Wolfgang Goethe-Universität
Robert-Mayer-Straße 5
Fach 107
D-60054 Frankfurt/M.
069 798 23889

Lightning Source UK Ltd.
Milton Keynes UK
24 March 2010

151839UK00002B/105/P

9 789042 026605